BREEDING BETTER DOGS

BREEDING BETTER DOGS

GENETICS AND REPRODUCTION

JULIE T. CECERE, DVM, MS, DACT

D. PHILLIP SPONENBERG, DVM, PHD, DACT

Virginia-Maryland College of Veterinary Medicine, Virginia Polytechnic
Institute and State University

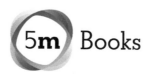

Published by
5M Books Ltd,
Lings, Great Easton,
Essex CM6 2HH, UK,
Tel +44 (0)330 1333 580
www.5mbooks.com

Follow us on
Twitter @5m_Books
Instagram 5m_books
Facebook @5mBooks
LinkedIn @5mbooks

A Catalogue record for this book is available from the British Library

ISBN 9781789182460
eISBN 9781789182613
DOI 10.52517/9781789182613

Book layout by Cheshire Typesetting Ltd, Cuddington, Cheshire
Printed by Hobbs the Printers
Photos by the authors unless otherwise indicated.

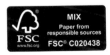

Contents

Preface

This book is the culmination of the authors' many decades of working directly with dog breeders as well as educating veterinarians. Those efforts have involved the details of the genetic side of dog breeding as well as the biologic details of canine reproduction, both of which are needed for dog breeders to succeed in producing top-quality dogs.

Many people have been helpful to both of us, and without their input this book would never have been possible. Acknowledgements always run the risk of overlooking some specific person, which must be kept in mind when any list of contributors is assembled. Despite the possibility of possible omissions, a handful of folks have been especially helpful to us.

Dr. Beverly Purswell stands out as having contributed greatly to the professional careers of both of us. Her detailed questions into the genetic management of breeds and kennels sparked many responses from Phil. She diligently educated Julie into the techniques and philosophies that lead to successful management of canine reproduction. Beverly has deeply contributed to both sides (genetic and reproductive) of dog breeding and has been essential in moving the field of canine breeding forward in many important ways.

Many other people have also helped this book to take its final form, especially by reading various chapters and offering substantive suggestions for improvement in clarity and presentation. Special thanks go to Laura Noll, Meredith Wadsworth, Heidi Phillips, Danielle Carpenter, and Nicole Sugai. Broad thanks also go out to our extensive contacts in the wide community of dog breeders. Without their support and contributions this book would not have been possible.

Any book has to go from the original idea and on through the writing and assembling figures. At that point it can seem almost finished, but much remains to be done before a final book emerges. The authors are both grateful and appreciative of the entire staff at 5m for their diligence in taking the book through those final essential steps. Working with the staff at 5m is always a delight. Their pleasant and constructive manner makes the process of going from manuscript to finished book enjoyable and productive.

CHAPTER 1

Breeding Dogs

This book delves into the many details around breeding dogs. The details can be broken down into two basic divisions:

- management and manipulation of genetics, including genes in specific matings as well as genes across entire populations such as kennels or breeds
- management of the biology of reproduction.

Proficiency in both is necessary for successful dog breeding (Figure 1.1).

This book is designed for various audiences. One audience is dog breeders, including those that are only beginning to consider breeding dogs, as well as those with multiple years of experience. Another audience is veterinarians in general practice. The most successful outcomes come when dog breeders and veterinarians combine their knowledge and skills to provide for a healthy and synergistic relationship that benefits all participants, including the dogs.

The specific cultural environment in which dog breeding occurs varies from region to region. Those differences are important because they influence much of what is possible for dog breeders to attain. Both authors reside in and work in the USA, where dog breeding has essentially no regulation at all by any governmental oversight. Despite this official lack of control, varying levels of influence are exercised by some American breed clubs or registries. The level of regulation varies but is usually only minimal or moderate in most cases.

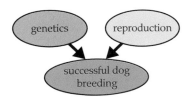

Figure 1.1 Successful dog breeding is the result of combining genetics with canine reproduction. Figure by DPS.

Because of the relative lack of formal breeding laws in the USA, decisions and actions of individual dog breeders often have minimal constraints there. Any progress in advancing the quality and health of dogs across the USA therefore relies on individual breeders and not on any other entity. Individual breeders that are educated and motivated are the key to success.

This book originates from that specific cultural background, and the relative lack of control in the USA is not true of the situation for breeders and veterinarians in some other regions or countries. The varying levels of external governance over dog breeding are an inherent limitation in a book such as this, although it remains true that targeting information to the "least regulated" situation does indeed help to deeply probe into general concepts. This can in turn help to generate sound and appropriate actions from within the community of breeders and veterinarians. The development of methods and approaches within the dog breeding community can actually lead to results that are more positive and longer lasting than would be possible if they were imposed by bodies outside the community.

This book aims to provide detailed discussions of a sequence of topics that are divided into chapters. The initial chapters consider the "genetics" of dog breeding with subsequential chapters progressing to the practical aspects of "dog reproduction". Each chapter presents detailed information that is then summarized by a brief list of key points that emphasize the main issues within the chapter that are most important to firmly grasp.

1.1 Why Dog Breeds?

The question "Why breed dogs?" is an important one, and for many people the answer is unfortunately less obvious today than it was a century ago. It may therefore be surprising to reverse that question to first ask "Why dog breeds?" Understanding the biology and function of dog breeds is an important basis for appreciating the value of dogs in today's world. This understanding can help to assure that the many benefits of dogs in society continue to be enjoyed for future generations of both dogs and their owners.

The importance and roles of dog breeds have recently undergone higher levels of scrutiny than those prevalent in past years. An unfortunate outcome of this scrutiny has been an increasing number of people now holding the view that purebred dog breeding is both problematic and detrimental to dog welfare. At a superficial level this can be true at least some of the time, but dog breeding done well can make essential and positive contributions to healthy, happy, and useful dogs that serve their owners well. Dogs and people can both gain immensely when dog selection and dog breeding are done well. Careful and insightful dog breeding is almost entirely undertaken only by those working within specific individual dog breeds.

Dogs have recently come to be seen as filling only one societal role, that of companion animals. Many random-bred and mixed breed dogs fill this niche and fill it well (although, to be fair, many do not!). This fact, combined with historic levels of dog over-population, has led many people to question the need for any purebred dogs, which has in turn led to the opposition to breeders and breeding of purebred dogs. This point of view often springs from a belief that there are already many dogs needing homes, so anyone who is deliberately planning to breed dogs is only contributing to a further increase in the problem of dog overpopulation.

In contrast to this view, there are many uses for dogs that still exist and that still need to be fulfilled on an ongoing basis. Many of the roles that dogs fulfill can only be accomplished by dogs that are capable of successfully performing very specific tasks. While currently only a minority of all dogs truly work for a living, these dogs are very essential components of the systems in which they serve. These roles include service dogs, search and rescue dogs, herding dogs, guarding dogs, a wide variety of hunting dogs, and a host of other very specific tasks for which some dogs are exquisitely well-suited while others can only perform poorly if at all. Dogs that are deliberately bred for a specific purpose are very likely to perform the desired task quite well, while nearly all other dogs are likely to be poorly suited for that task. The right dog in the right role is a joy to watch as it works (Figure 1.2). The wrong dog in the wrong role can cause never-ending headaches and are only rarely able to fully achieve the specific goals.

Dogs that are purposely bred to perform specific jobs are essential in those roles. This by no means diminishes the important role useful and often essential role for dogs as the "companion animal" (Figure 1.3). While the role of companion animal might be simplistically seen as an easy role for nearly any dog, the truth is that not all dogs perform equally well in all companion situations. A variable pool of candidate dogs is a valuable asset in this case, because ideally each individual dog comes with its own predictable array of character traits that help to assure a good match of dog, owner, and setting. The best dog for a rambunctious eight-year-old boy is very likely to be different than the dog best suited to an elderly woman living alone.

The link between dog and job is where purpose-bred, purebred dogs enter the picture. An essential key to the usefulness of pure dog breeds is the predictability of their characteristics such as behavioral tendencies, body type, proportion, size, coat type, and color, most of which are described in the breed standards. It can be more difficult to appreciate the broader contributions that a breed's genetic package makes to temperament and behavioral traits that are even more important on a daily basis than the more obvious superficial traits. A purebred dog should have "the whole package" of its breed – both the external and the internal components. The repeatability of the breed package assures that dogs can partner with their owners in a predictable and positive way. Having distinct breeds of dogs

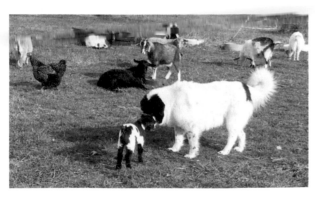

Figure 1.2 Livestock guardian dogs, like this Karakachan dog, are an essential tool for small ruminant production in most parts of the world. The calm demeanor of the goats and chickens indicates that this individual dog is a good fit for this role. Photo by DPS.

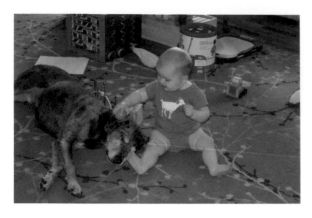

Figure 1.3 Safe and dependable companion dogs serve their families well and contribute greatly to human well-being, while also enjoying safe and secure lives themselves. Photo by JTC.

brings great value to dog use and enjoyment. An array of unique breeds allows prospective owners to select a dog that best meets their own individual needs and desires.

The predictability of the package of traits for each breed comes from relative genetic uniformity that is shared among the members of the breed. Even within a group of related breeds that are used for similar purposes, the tailoring of the breed package for a specific task is a balancing act that can take the final dog in different directions. For example, within the group of Retrievers are several breeds, each with a slightly different array of preferred approaches to the task, and each of which is a more logical fit for some situations than for others. Individual breeds are therefore important, even within a group of related breeds used for similar purposes. A lack of predictability makes it impossible for owners to choose a dog that is most likely to meet their specific needs, so some level of genetic uniformity is essential.

Dog breeds have achieved their status as predictable genetic resources by a combination of foundation, isolation, and selection (Figure 1.4). These three basic factors interact in different ways in each breed, but it is important that breeders understand all of these factors so that they can manage dog breeds for maximum long-term success.

The term "Foundation" refers to the specific dogs that were part of the original population from which the breed descends. Most of the early variation among dog breeds was shaped largely by geography and the chance events that took dogs from place to place with

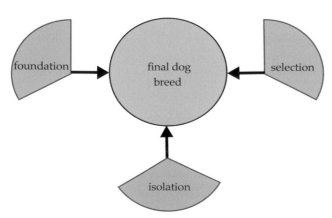

Figure 1.4 Each dog breed relies on its unique combination of foundation, genetic isolation, and selection to achieve its final form and function. Figure by DPS.

their human owners. Local dogs were mated together and then the offspring were selected for specific purposes whether that be livestock guardians, hunting dogs of various sorts, herding dogs, companion dogs, or others. The specific foundation population constrains the final form of the dogs that descend from it to be within a certain range. Basically, it is difficult or impossible to pull something out of a pot if it is not already in there somewhere by virtue of being included in the foundation.

A good example of the powerful influence of foundation on the final breed product comes from the large group of northern breeds loosely grouped together as Spitz dogs. These dogs all share a similar body type despite huge differences in size as well as in function. Some of these breeds serve as draft dogs for pulling, others function as hounds, others are herding dogs, and many more are companion dogs (Figure 1.5). These differences in ability are all imposed by selection on an originally somewhat limited foundation, a foundation that constrains the final product to be within certain boundaries and that can easily be recognized as "Spitz."

Following the foundation of a genetic population of dogs, genetic isolation helps to achieve relative uniformity of the population's genetic material. In past centuries, the isolation of dog breeds was largely due to geographical constraints as well as the culture within the breeder community that shared common goals, mentored younger breeders, and eventually established registries. This situation imposes human control over which individual dog mates with which other dog and assures some degree of isolation of genetic material. The final step in the process of genetically isolating dog breeds involved the establishment of formal registries. These have a practice of limiting registration of purebred dogs to those that have parents that are both of the same breed. Isolation prevents new and unusual genetic variants from entering the breed, and in that sense keeps the breed predictable in regard to the original breed package.

The details of isolation vary, with a tendency for breeds to become ever more isolated from one another as time progresses. This has varying causes. One such cause is simply historic, as illustrated by the livestock guard dogs from Eastern Europe. Shepherds in the Balkans a few centuries ago were part of the Ottoman Empire, and internal national

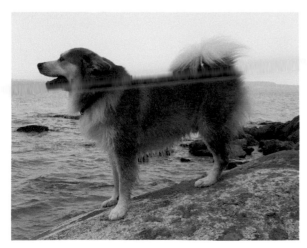

Figure 1.5 The Icelandic Sheepdog has a general shape and body style that reflects its Spitz origins, while its function as a herding dog reflects centuries of selection for specific behavioral traits and ability. Photo by Stuart Marsh.

boundaries did not exist within it. Shepherds, and their guard dogs, from the region that is now separated into Greece, Bulgaria, Macedonia, and Albania, might well all have been spending summers on the same mountain ranges. Their guard dogs would then have been a somewhat fluid single population due to these contacts. More firmly established national boundaries came after the end of World War I, which disrupted historic seasonal migrations with its opportunities for genetic exchanges. As a result, each national population of livestock guardian dogs has become increasingly distinct due to the isolation imposed by the political boundaries and the movement of people, dogs, and sheep.

A similar outcome, from a different starting point, is the small "earth dog" terrier breeds that were sequentially pulled out of the general "hunt terrier" population (Figure 1.6). Breeders of these "earth dogs" across different locations emphasized slightly different traits and as these populations became increasingly isolated, they were well on their way to becoming distinct breeds within this more general group. Most breeds of coonhounds in North America share a similar trajectory: sequential isolation from what was once a single, more variable, population.

Selection is the final component of breed formation. Selection simply means that some dogs reproduce, and others do not, and that matings between specific individual dogs are planned out by their owners. Human owners almost entirely control purebred dog reproduction. Selection is a powerful tool and has historically been used to shape the function of dogs as well as their external looks. Selection has powerful consequences for the final product and must therefore be done wisely and with a comprehensive view of the desired final purebred dog. Selection must always strike a balance between ability and looks because both are critically important for breed maintenance. Ability is more difficult to assess than looks but remains an essential target of selection.

The interaction of foundation, isolation, and selection varies from breed to breed. Of these three, isolation and selection have become the most powerful influences across most

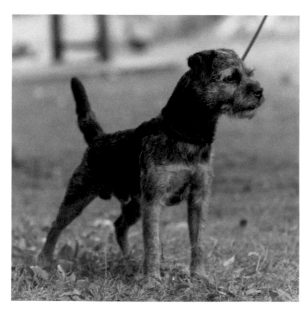

Figure 1.6 Small terriers, including Border Terriers, are a group of breeds that come from a similar gene pool. Photo by Jasmine Sanders.

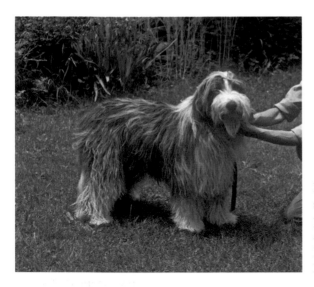

Figure 1.7 Selection has powerfully shaped the Bearded Collie into the present-day breed that springs from an original foundation shared by other herding dogs in the United Kingdom. Photo by DPS.

dog breeds today. The foundation of most dog breeds was established many decades, or even centuries, ago and the exact details are often incompletely known. With a few exceptions, foundation cannot be changed. Complete isolation is currently the general rule for purebred dog breeding, which limits genetic variation to what is available at every generational step. For most breeds, foundation and isolation are firmly set in place, and dog breeding must continue within the limits imposed by these two.

In contrast, selection is an ongoing factor (Figure 1.7). This makes selection the most powerful current influence of the three because it is the one factor that current breeders can control. Breeders can change which specific traits are of interest or can pursue (or avoid) certain specific bloodlines or individual dogs within a breed. Changes in selection influence the underlying breed package, and therefore must be undertaken wisely. Selection must carefully consider what is practical and will lead to long-term viability and success for the breed.

For many of today's dog breeds, an important stage of breed development is best captured by the concept of "gentrification." This term was proposed by David Nelson, a longtime breeder of Kangal and Akbash dogs. Gentrification has influences from foundation, isolation, and selection. A breed is taken from its original homeland, imported somewhere else, and is then selected for a use other than the original purpose. This imposes a sort of "secondary foundation" that is often much more restricted than the original one that was present in the homeland. The resulting breed therefore contains less variation than the larger population from which it was originally pulled, and in many cases also includes various genetic or structural weaknesses that need to be addressed. While less variation means more uniformity and more predictability, it can also lead to less viability when levels of variability become too low or when weaknesses emerge that were hidden in the foundation stock. The gentrification process is the history behind most dog breeds today, and most often this has occurred in Europe. A good example is the Afghan hound, essential for hunting in Afghanistan but rarely used for that purpose in Europe or North America where the breed has been standardized for the show ring after importation from its homeland.

The cascade of foundation, isolation, and selection can have interesting consequences over time. The herding dogs of the United Kingdom are a good example. Centuries ago, these were variable dogs with a wide range of coat types, colors, and working styles. From that common foundation, today's breeds have been formed by isolation and selection for use in situations that varied by topography and animal management practices. That process has given us the Border Collie, Bearded Collie, Collie (further separated into Rough and Smooth), Old English Sheepdog, Welsh Sheepdog, Shetland Sheepdog, English Shepherd, Australian Cattle Dog, and others. At least one breed from this group, the Patagonian Sheepdog, is an early offshoot of the foundation population that has somehow managed to maintain a great deal of the underlying genetic variation that has been lost in the other breeds as they have split off from the original larger group (Figure 1.8). The breeds within this group demonstrate the process of breed formation through foundation, followed by isolation, and then finally tailored by selection that splits dogs into isolated breeds each serving a specific purpose and having a specific appearance.

Dog breeds are distinctive from one another. Dogs of most breeds cannot be easily mistaken for another breed, even though a few exceptions to this rule do occur. Beneath the level of "breed" are other divisions, such as varieties and bloodlines. Varieties are usually single-gene differences in traits such as coat type. Collies, for example, come in two varieties based on their haircoat: rough and smooth. Dachshunds sport three varieties: shorthaired, longhaired, and wirehaired. The approach of splitting out varieties varies from region to region and can lead to increasing levels of isolation of one variety from another. One example comes from the Belgian sheep herding breeds. In the USA, each color or coat type is considered a separate breed, while in Europe they are all considered one breed with the consequence that mating among the various varieties is acceptable (Figure 1.9).

Bloodlines are a more subtle method of division than varieties. Bloodlines include dogs that are generally more related to one another than they are to other dogs within the

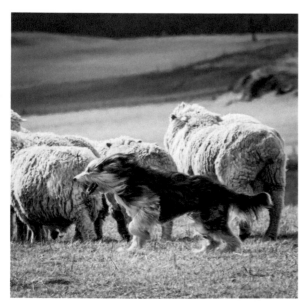

Figure 1.8 The Patagonian Sheepdog retains a broader genetic variation than other breeds of herding dogs that originated in the United Kingdom. Photo by Natasha Barrios.

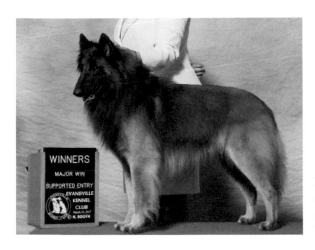

Figure 1.9 The Belgian herding dogs are all considered one breed in Belgium but are separated out by color varieties in the USA. Photo by Connie Perdue.

same breed. Bloodlines do not always have clean crisp borders that separate them from one another. Despite their somewhat loose definition, bloodlines are still an important way to partition the genetics of a breed.

Bloodlines fall into somewhat broader divisions based on type in some breeds. "Type" in this sense can be equated with "breed type," which is the combination of general build, body shape, coat, head character, and behavioral traits that characterize a dog breed. The final type of dog, or group of dogs, depends a great deal on selection. Many hunting breeds have a field trial type as well as a show type. Other breeds have distinct types based on region of origin, with many breeds having a different type in Europe than in the United States.

The different types within a single breed can be so distinct from one another that they are rarely mated together because the result would be combinations that are poorly suited to either of the end uses. The extent of the separation raises the very important question of "what is a breed?" because in an extreme case the complete isolation of types can easily lead to what are essentially two breeds that have complete genetic isolation from each other. Each of these "daughter breeds" springs from a single foundation in the earlier breed but then has been separated out by isolation from the other as well as by selection for the relevant differences in function and looks.

Informed breeders are sensitive to all these details of how breeds were developed and how they are maintained. The decisions of individual breeders figure into this broader picture and need to be carefully considered if the goal is the long-term maintenance of the breed. Once this is understood, it is possible for breeders at all levels to engage more fully in dog breeding and in breed maintenance.

An essential first step for knowledgeable breeders is for them to understand their own breed and their own dogs. It is important for breeders to sort through some of the mythology around their own breed to arrive at a clear-headed appreciation for the breed and for the potential it has for useful function.

The detailed ways in which dog breeds differ from one another are important parts of why each breed fits into a specific role for its owners. Breed history and breed use are both important because these reflect the genetic hard wiring that makes specific breeds ideal for specific tasks, while also being a very poor fit for others. No single breed can do it all, despite many overly optimistic breed descriptions that are easily encountered and that can mislead people new to dogs or new to specific dog breeds.

Most breeds share some overlap of characteristics such as foundation, type, and function with at least a few other breeds. This leads to the idea of "breed groups" although the criteria used to decide the specific group to which a breed belongs can vary from country to country.

The viewpoint of "groups of breeds with similar uses" is practical and constructive, but it is important to remember that breed groups commonly used by kennel clubs do not always coincide with breed groupings that are based on biology, behavior, and use. At least some of the groupings used by kennel clubs have been historically more related to the organization of dog shows than they were to any other purpose. This approach can group some breeds together that have very little in common with one another. The key point to understand is that breeds with similar purposes almost always have similar genetic potential to accomplish that purpose, and often share relationships from a similar foundation.

A good example of the need for clear-headed appreciation of breed groups comes from the "working dogs" group that includes several different breeds. Within this large group are livestock guardians, which work best when prey drive is weak or absent. In contrast, many of the other breeds in the working group are not livestock guardians at all and have a fairly high prey drive. Dogs from those breeds cannot be expected to perform the livestock guardian task well, if at all, even though they are all considered "working breeds."

Another pitfall relates to breed descriptions, and the herding breed group illustrates this well. Some breed descriptions indicate that the breed shows both herding and guarding behavior (Figure 1.10). In this case, "guarding" can include two different aspects. One is bonding to and guarding livestock, which is generally a behavior opposite to what is needed in a herding dog because a good herding dog has prey drive while a good livestock

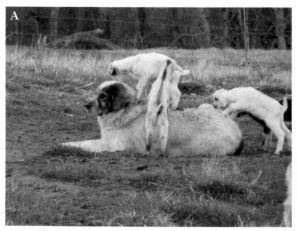 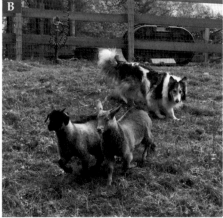

Figure 1.10 A: Livestock guardians should have little or no prey drive to most effectively do their job. Their charges do not respond to them as they would to a predator. B: In contrast, herding dogs like the Old-Time Scotch Collie rely on prey drive to control and manipulate livestock. Photo A by DPS, Photo B by Leslie Allen.

guardian lacks this. A second sort of guarding relates to facilities and people, a task that is easily accomplished by a herding dog. Very few dogs can do all three tasks: herding, guarding livestock, and guarding premises. If people are seeking such a dog based off an overly optimistic breed description, they are likely to be sorely disappointed by most candidates! How a dog accomplishes its task often involves some level of genetic hard-wiring, and it is essential to consider this when matching a breed to a situation. It is important to accurately define the task that needs to be done, and then to match the right dog from the right breed with that task.

The average ability of dogs within a single breed to accomplish a specific task can be a useful guide to breed selection. However, within the averages across a single breed, individual dogs within a breed, or even within a single litter, vary in the degree to which they have the genetic machinery for a specific behavior or task. Some of the abilities can be assessed relatively early in life, others are only evident at maturity or with appropriate training. Assessing differences that are evident early in life can help to place individual dogs in appropriate situations so that they can excel. Early evaluations need to be followed by ongoing attention to individual details of behavior and ability as they become evident throughout the dog's life. These later evaluations build upon early decisions as dogs progress to adulthood. All these details are extremely important in guiding final decisions as to which specific dogs to mate together, which then produce the next generation of the breed.

Mating two dogs together that are both from the same extreme end of a breed's distribution of physical traits, temperament, or behavior nearly assures the production of puppies that are all at that same extreme end. While this sounds harmless, the extreme in some situations can end up being too much of a good thing. "More" can end up being "too much" instead of "just enough." This circles back to selection, and to the ongoing need for selection to be wise, balanced, and targeted at long-term goals for the breed.

1.2 Why Breed Dogs?

People embark on the journey of dog breeding for a whole host of reasons, some of which are more productive than others. Basic reasons for wanting to breed dogs should be carefully considered. Having a deep appreciation for an individual's reasons for breeding dogs greatly helps to chart out goals for the breeding program. Many of the reasons that lie behind a decision to breed dogs lead to constructive and positive outcomes. Reasons that are deliberate and well-thought can work to effectively guide a breeding program. Reasons and goals help to shape much of the decision-making that goes into breeding sound, healthy dogs that can then provide their owners with years of satisfying companionship, work, or service. In contrast, breeding operations that lack deliberate thought and decision-making often make little progress, and rarely produce excellent dogs.

Dog breeding has a cast of four main central characters: the dog, the breeder, the breed, and the puppy buyer. It is all too common for the role and stake of one or more of these to be diminished or even overlooked completely (Figure 1.11). The four main participants in a dog breeding program each have an important stake in the outcome. The needs of all four need to be carefully considered so that a successful breeding program can work to the benefit of all involved. Carelessly planned programs can easily do great damage to one or

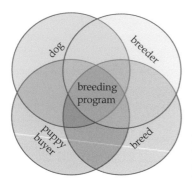

Figure 1.11 A breeding program is where the interests of the breeder, the dog, the breed, and puppy buyers all intersect. Figure by DPS.

more of these central participants, with the prospective puppy buyer in an especially vulnerable position. The potential damage, and reasons for it, need to be explored to increase awareness of potential pitfalls.

One obvious member of the team is the dog breeder. It makes little sense for a dog breeding program to adversely affect the breeder involved, whether that is financially, emotionally, or both. Relationships with puppy buyers can influence this aspect greatly because high demand for puppies eliminates the possibility of unsold puppies being retained by the breeder despite having limited potential in their own breeding program. Strategic goals that are not carefully thought out can evolve and change in subtle ways that can lead to significant damage to the breeder. No breeder sets out to do self-harm, but motivations can change over time and can lead to a very negative outcome. One reasonably common negative outcome relates to an unplanned increase in the size and complexity of a breeding operation. What began as an environment where all participants benefitted can become one with too many dogs, too little money, and too little time. In this situation it is common to lose the close and positive bond between the breeder and the dogs that characterized the early years of the endeavor. The breeder loses both emotionally and financially.

The dogs themselves are also involved in a breeding program. They have a huge stake in the outcome, despite having very little direct control over goals and decisions. Programs that produce dogs that are successful in their roles are highly valued. Successful dogs are viable, and their functional success should be easily achieved through reasonable levels of training. This sort of dog is highly appreciated by its owners, and relationships between such dogs and their owners are great examples of good and positive human-animal bonds. However, it is easy to forget or downplay the role and risk of individual dogs in a breeding program. They can too easily become mere game-pieces to be manipulated and exploited. The most extreme example is commercial "puppy mills" where dogs are kept confined in small spaces and whose only function is their reproductive contribution to the endeavor. Dogs deserve better than that! It is ideal that dogs used in a breeding program are themselves integral components of constructive and positive situations with their humans, whether those are based on companionship or on services that the dogs provide. The idea of partnership cannot be overemphasized because it is where dogs and people benefit the most.

The dog breed itself is also an important participant in dog breeding endeavors. The role played by the dog breed is a bit more nebulous than the previous two but is equally important if long-term success is to be achieved. Dog breeding should benefit the breed, and this can take on many different dimensions. A breeding program should leave the breed in better genetic condition than when it began. This is a complicated issue, and no single approach is going to be best in all situations. Strong breeding programs produce good dogs that build demand for the breeder's dogs, and for the breed. Beneath that broad umbrella are a host of issues that vary from breed to breed, requiring specific recommendations that are closely tailored to individual situations.

Puppy buyers influence all the other main participants in many ways. They create the demand that keeps a breeder in a secure situation. Demand also tends to put individual dogs in situations that are appropriate, whether that be in a breeding program, a companion situation, or as a working partner. Buyers can also be important sources of monitoring the general health of both individual dogs and the breed because they can observe the dog over its entire lifetime.

A few reasons for breeding dogs stand out as lacking significant long-term contributions to the interests of dogs, breeders, and breeds. One reason that is sometimes put forward is "so the children can see the miracle of birth." This is not inherently wrong, but it does put minimal emphasis on several of the participants. The breeding dogs involved likely have a pretty decent situation. The resulting litter of puppies, though, may not all find homes where they will be well cared for and highly valued. Contributions to the breeder's life can also be minimal. And, with a few exceptions, any potential long-term contribution to the breed involved is also minimized.

"Making money" is another reason for some people that endeavor to breed dogs. Some breeders do indeed make money through breeding dogs, but there are easier ways to make money! Breeding operations that emphasize monetary return often involve many dogs. As breeding operations scale up, problems tend to increase in severity and frequency so that the final profitability of the whole endeavor tends to lag. This is especially true when considering the time and resources that are required for success. This usually occurs in situations where the operation's size precludes adequate animal care and management. Animal assessment is important in any breeding program and is often the first aspect to be dropped when a breeding program's size becomes unmanageable. Talented, organized, and thoughtful breeders can indeed manage a large and profitable breeding program, but it takes planning and hard work. And, if monetary concerns are driving the enterprise, it often works out that the dogs involved have at least a somewhat substandard life. This can also be true for the puppies that are produced. Short-term concerns for profitability often minimize any long-term positive outcomes for the breed involved.

Some breeders deliberately pursue the production and campaigning of show winning dogs (Figure 1.12). A host of different motivations can lie behind this desire, with important differences between shows, performance trials, or other competitive situations. Each of these has its own set of criteria and procedures for participation. Breeders seeking to succeed in these activities pay careful attention to the type and style of the dogs involved and target their breeding programs to take advantage of what is currently being rewarded in whichever of these various events they have targeted. Breeders can benefit greatly from participation, not only in general terms of lifestyle but also financially. The dogs can also benefit, with the caution that in some cases these competitions can favor extremes of type

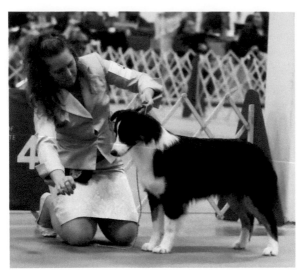

Figure 1.12 Showing dogs is a popular endeavor that can either help or harm dogs and dog breeds. Photo by JTC.

or behavior, some of which are not always in the dog's, owner's, or breed's best interest long-term.

The consequences of breeding programs that target the production of winners can be subtle and complex for breeds. These are often somewhat negative because fewer and fewer dogs participate in producing the next generation of the breed because breeders chase after the dogs that are currently winning, and then use them heavily. That situation can collapse the genetic variation that is so necessary for any breed's long-term successful future.

Breeders should always consider what specific contributions they are making to the breed. Some breeders choose to work with a specific bloodline to mold it and assure its overall quality and soundness. Other breeders choose to specifically work with rare breeds. Projects with rare breeds bring with them a host of challenges. Breeding programs for rare breeds require a lot of planning and attention to detail because decisions need to keep long-term consequences in mind. These go well into the future and many of the consequences are not particularly obvious in the short term. Rare breeds benefit most greatly by having increased numbers, broader distribution, and a healthy genetic situation both in terms of population structure, as well as regarding genetic defects. Some of these more constructive aspects can be missing from programs that are based on interest in the breed only for its novelty.

Some breeders are fascinated by the puzzle of being able to put the genetic pieces together to lead to new varieties or variations in a specific breed. The results of this sort of motivation vary greatly, from very positive to very negative. The most negative extreme can find the dogs only valued for their ability to contribute to the final desired combination of traits. Such dogs might find only limited use for a short period, and then they might be shunted off to fairly substandard lives. In addition, overall balance and soundness can be sacrificed in the quest for the expression of some traits that are found only in those few dogs that carry them. Avid pursuit of certain rare combinations can downplay the overall soundness and vitality of the dogs involved. This is especially likely when fads promote certain rare colors or other traits of cosmetic rather than function.

In contrast, putting the various components together in a sound and serviceable final canine form can be very rewarding for all involved. This involves careful consideration of a whole host of issues, and the challenge can be an intriguing undertaking for a dedicated breeder. The complex interaction of breeder, dog, and breed comes into play, and managing these constructively and successfully can be immensely rewarding.

These are only a handful of the many motivations that can lie behind a breeding program. While any one of these can predominate, it is also common for them to be combined in various ways. Potential dog breeders should reflect on their motivations and set goals, and then acquire the tools and education to meet those goals. Goals, and the means to achieve them, are essential if progress is to be made. Blending the major motivations in various ways can be very effective in setting goals that will lead to an enjoyable and successful program with benefits to all involved.

1.3 Key Points

- Successful dog breeders are knowledgeable about genetics as well as dog reproduction.
- Pure dog breeds are important because they are predictable.
- The predictability of dog breeds provides for an effective match of dog and situation.
- Predictability needs to be safeguarded for the long-term future.
- Dog breeders have an essential role in safeguarding dog breeds as viable genetic resources.
- The best dog breeders have specific goals for long-term success.
- Good breeding programs have positive outcomes for dog breeds, dog breeders, individual dogs, and puppy buyers.

CHAPTER 2

Genetic Tools for Breeders

Breeders have a variety of tools at their disposal. Each of them contributes in a different way to a successful breeding program that produces sound and useful dogs. The many tools can be sorted into two main divisions:

- genetic management strategies for populations and individuals
- biology and management of reproduction.

The genetic side of the breeding program provides the basic foundation for the production of sound dogs and sound breeds. To that foundation a breeder must add the biologic aspects of reproduction, without which the genetics tools cannot succeed. Genetics only works if a next generation is coming along! The next few chapters of this book delve into the "genetics" portion of the toolkit. This chapter deals mostly with the tools, followed by chapters on how they can be used effectively in a breeding program. The genetics information is followed by the "reproduction" side of the tool kit in succeeding chapters.

2.1 Basics of Genetics

Dogs are highly variable in size, coat, color, behavior, and a host of other characteristics. Most of this variation originates in variation of the underlying genetics that control these traits. Genetic control is most readily grasped for obviously expressed traits such as coat color, but genetic control is also behind the more subtle or complicated traits like ability, conformation, and temperament. A general understanding of genetics, and how to use genetic information, is a necessary underpinning for making progress toward any goal in dog breeding.

Genes contribute to an individual dog's well-being, as well as to the security of a breed. Understanding how genetic information functions and how it flows from generation to generation can help breeders to achieve good outcomes. Breeders gain the most from genetics when they approach it seriously, but also with imagination and creativity. It is important to remember that genetics is a "power tool." When used wisely and appropriately, it can help get a lot of work done and done well. When used poorly, it can result in great damage and can do so very quickly.

The science of genetics can be unnerving to many people but is greatly simplified when a few key rules are remembered. Most of the confusion surrounding genetics comes from the words used, rather than the concepts that those words represent. Understanding a few basic concepts greatly simplifies navigating the details of any genetic system. Although the following discussion simplifies some details, it should provide a basic understanding that can be used in practical ways to help dog breeders achieve their goals. It begins with the definitions of several basic terms, each of which means something very specific. Understanding these definitions helps to improve and facilitate accurate communication among breeders, customers, and veterinarians.

"Phenotype" is an important term that refers to any characteristic of an organism. In dogs these include external features such as conformation, coat type, and color. They also include more complex features such as functional traits, temperament, and behavioral tendencies. An animal's phenotype results from the interaction of an animal's genetic makeup (known as their "genotype") and the many environmental factors that act on and influence it (Figure 2.1). The final phenotype observed in a dog, therefore, may or may not accurately reveal all aspects of its genotype.

Breeders are usually most interested in the genotype of an animal. Genotypes are often determined with genetic testing, but many traits can also be accurately documented by direct observation or knowledge of parental traits. A dog's genotype is of special interest to breeders as it determines the offspring's range of potential genotypes, and therefore final phenotypes. This in turn determines the basic breeding value of that individual dog. Making a link between phenotype and genotype is the goal of genetics, because ensuring healthy and appropriate genotypes is the surest way to produce desirable phenotypes in the offspring. The environmental influences that interact with the genotype to produce the final phenotype can complicate the complete expression of the genotype in various ways. In some cases, this interaction is favorable and leads to strongly positive outcomes. In other cases, the interaction can be negative with less favorable outcomes being produced. Regardless of the outcomes, the fact remains that the environment can only influence what is already present in the genotype, so it is the genotype that realistically sets the limit on potential phenotypes.

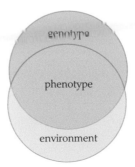

Figure 2.1 The interaction of genes and environment shapes the final phenotype of a dog. The management of this interaction is important to the outcome. Figure by DPS.

Dogs, perhaps more than most other species, have final phenotypes that are profoundly affected by the combination of genotype and environmental influences. This is especially true for traits that relate to working functions like hunting prowess, athletic ability, and guarding ability. Behavioral traits such as trainability and basic temperament are likewise shaped by a profound interaction between the genotype and environmental influences. Most of the behavioral ability that a dog has, and that contributes to a good match with specific purposes, is shaped strongly by environmental influences, such as socialization and training. Many of the environmental influences are time-sensitive, and several are limited to certain periods of the dog's development.

Importantly, the genetic contributions and the environmental contributions (training and socialization) each have complete veto over success in the final product (Figure 2.2). Both are essential and need to be appropriate to the final use and function of the specific dog in its specific role. A lack of either can result in the overall failure in the ability of the dog to serve its intended purpose.

Despite the importance of environmental influences, shaping genotypes is the first step in producing the base from which a good and useful dog can be produced. It is also the aspect of the whole process over which breeding decisions have the most influence. Remember, though, that the best genetic package can be mishandled, and this can still lead to failure. On the other side of the coin, the worst genetic package cannot be made successful even with the best management and training. Genetics establishes the potential of the dog, after which the environment shapes this potential into the final product.

Genetic information controls the wide array of traits in dogs and occurs as discrete and repeatable pieces. These pieces of information are made of deoxyribonucleic acid (DNA) and are known as genes. Each gene generally controls a specific trait, in a one-to-one relationship. Genes are organized sequentially along structures called chromosomes. Dogs have 78 chromosomes in the nucleus of each cell (except for mature

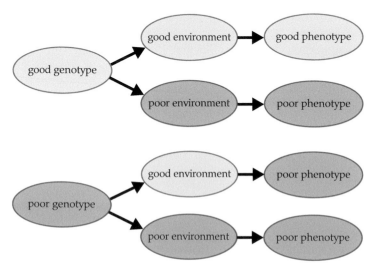

Figure 2.2 Due to the complete veto of genotype and environment, good final phenotypes depend on both being optimal. Figure by DPS.

red blood cells) and these chromosomes consist of 39 pairs. This is a highly organized system in which each individual gene has a specific site on a specific chromosome. This arrangement influences the way the genes operate and are transmitted from generation to generation.

Generally, both members of a chromosome pair have identical sequences of genes. One exception to this general rule is the pair of chromosomes known as the sex chromosomes, which determine the sex of the animal. The specific function of the sex chromosomes is related to the fact that the two types of sex chromosomes do not have identical sequences of genes. Fortunately, the genetic information on the sex chromosomes is important in only a few situations aside from sex determination. In those few situations, though, the sex chromosomes become very important indeed. This is the basis of "sex linkage" of some traits because they pass along the generations associated with one sex or the other due to their location on a sex chromosome.

A useful, but somewhat oversimplified, way to picture chromosomes is to imagine a sequence of beads (genes) on a string (chromosome) (Figure 2.3). The genes on each chromosome exist in a specific highly ordered arrangement that repeats across all dogs. The specific location of a gene is known as its locus. A locus, therefore, is a sort of address for the physical site of a gene within the genetic material. The plural of locus is loci.

The loci are all neatly and orderly arranged along the chromosomes, but the specific information in genetic material at those loci often varies among individual dogs. This is the underlying source of variability in the final traits that each dog expresses. These changes occur in a process called mutation, which produces alternate forms of the original genetic code. The various forms of a gene are called alleles and include the original form as well as each different mutation. The cause of this variability includes several different mechanisms:

- single-point differences in the DNA sequence
- duplications of portions of the DNA sequence
- deletions of portions of the DNA sequence
- insertions of portions from other lengths of DNA.

The most common sort of mutation is a single-point change in the DNA sequence. DNA is made of biochemical units called nucleotides, so this sort of mutation is called a single-nucleotide polymorphism (SNP). Deletions or duplications of portions of the DNA can also result from mutations, as can insertion of a length of DNA into a sequence where it did not originally occur.

The importance of these mutations is that a single locus can have many different

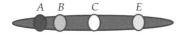

Figure 2.3 Chromosomes can be viewed somewhat simplistically as tightly ordered specific sequences of genetic loci that line up like beads on a string. Each locus has its own specific spot on a specific chromosome. Figure by DPS.

alleles. However, each individual dog can only have up to two alleles at any one locus. This is because each dog only has two copies of each gene due to the paired character of the chromosomes. One slight modification to this simplistic view is that a few important traits are governed by situations where an entire gene has been duplicated and is therefore present as more than the usual two copies. These are rare in dogs and can generally be ignored.

The alleles at a specific locus can interact in different ways. One of these is dominance, the other side of which is recessiveness. Dominant alleles are expressed equally well in the phenotype whether the dominant allele is present as only one copy of the pair, or as both copies. Recessive alleles, in contrast, are only expressed in the phenotype if both copies of the pair are the same. Dominant alleles mask recessive alleles when they are paired together, so in this situation the recessive allele is unexpressed (hidden). Importantly, this means that the expression of the recessive allele (or gene, these two words are often used interchangeably) can pop up as a surprise. This occurs (in a minority of offspring) when the recessive allele becomes paired with another copy of the same allele following the mating of two animals that both carry that same recessive allele. Dominance is therefore one mechanism by which a portion of the genome is hidden from expression. The recessive allele is still present, and can still be passed along, but it is hidden from view in the phenotype by virtue of being masked by the presence of the dominant allele. The concept that portions of the genome can be hidden is an important one, and dominance is one of the common mechanisms behind this.

Most discussions of genes resort to convenient abbreviated symbols for alleles. One common practice is to use capital symbols for dominant alleles, and lower-case symbols for recessive alleles. These are often in italics to emphasize that they are symbols. "A" is a dominant allele, "a" is a recessive allele. Some loci have more than two alleles, so this convenient and simple solution does not work for all loci. To get around that problem, one solution is to always include a locus symbol, with the allele abbreviation as a superscript. By this system, the capital letter designates a specific locus, and the superscript designates a specific allele at that locus.

This system of symbols works well for loci that have more than two alleles. This includes many loci. At these loci the alleles can have complex interactions, with some alleles being dominant, some recessive, and some intermediate or variable depending on the specific pair of alleles that is present. One example is the *Agouti* locus, where "A^Y" is a dominant allele for sable color, "A^t" is an intermediate allele that results in black and tan color (recessive to A^Y but dominant to A^a), and "A^a" is a recessive allele that leads to a fairly rare recessive black color. The key point is that each allele is potentially dominant (or recessive) to others and understanding this aspect of the specific allele of interest is the key to managing it in breeding decisions.

Different genetic testing companies use different abbreviations for alleles, but most of them are reasonably easy to understand. The important detail is to know which abbreviation or symbol correlates to which allele, and then to understand how those alleles interact when paired together.

The term homozygous is used to describe a pair of alleles that are identical. This is true whether the gene is dominant or recessive, the term only refers to the fact that both copies

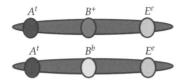

Figure 2.4 Chromosomes are paired, so genetic loci are also paired. The presence of identical alleles, or of different alleles, at each locus is important. In this example, the *A* and *E* loci are homozygous, both members of the pair are the same, and therefore only that one allele can be passed on to the offspring. In contrast, the *B* locus is heterozygous, and the animal can pass along either allele to its offspring.

are the same. Homozygous animals can obviously only pass along that one allele to their offspring. In contrast, the term heterozygous refers to a pair containing two different alleles for the same gene. Animals with a heterozygous pair of alleles can pass along either allele to their offspring (Figure 2.4).

Importantly, the concept of dominance and recessiveness only describes the interaction of two alleles at a single locus. It does not relate at all to the frequency of the alleles in a breed. "Frequency" specifically refers to how often each allele occurs in the population being considered. Some breeds are uniform for recessive alleles, such as the liver color of German Shorthaired Pointers. Some breeds have dominant alleles that are relatively rare in the breed, such as the merle allele in Dachshunds that produces the dapple color in that breed.

It is important to not confuse allele frequency with dominance. The status of an allele as dominant or recessive does not change over time, even though its frequency can. Even if a recessive allele is uniform throughout a breed (the chocolate color of Boykin spaniels, for instance) it is still recessive. This becomes obvious in crossbred offspring where the expression of a recessive allele becomes hidden if the other parent breed has a dominant allele at the same locus.

Two important concepts involve situations that are intermediate between the usual dominant-or-recessive pattern. These are codominance and incomplete dominance, and they function slightly differently from one another.

Codominance occurs when both alleles in the pair are expressed. In a sense, neither is dominating the other, but both are expressed. Codominance is very common in the expression of proteins such as those that are important in blood types, but fairly rare in genetic systems that lead to easily visible manifestations. These are systems where the individual protein forms of each allele can be expressed fully, and they are usually measured by laboratory tests and cannot be detected by external examination of more obvious features.

Incomplete dominance is slightly different. It occurs where two, one, or no copies of an allele each have a different and recognizable result in the appearance of the animal. In most cases of incomplete dominance each homozygote has a specific appearance. The heterozygote usually has an appearance intermediate between the two different homozygotes (Figure 2.5). This can be thought of as three levels of expression of the same basic trait, in contrast to codominance where both alleles are expressed reasonably fully.

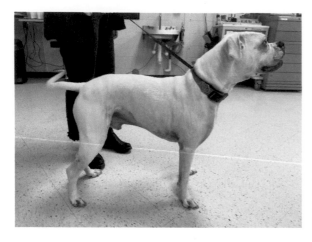

Figure 2.5 White Boxers are most consistently produced from mating two Boxers with white collar markings. Photo by JTC.

One example of incomplete dominance is one of the alleles that adds white to a Boxer dog's color. Dogs with no copies of the allele are the usual Boxer with minimal white on the legs, belly, and lower neck. Dogs with one copy of the allele have a greater amount of white, usually including a broad white band around the neck. Dogs with two copies of the allele are white or nearly so. Another example is the merle allele. Dogs that are homozygous for the normal allele are uniformly dark colored, while those homozygous for the merle allele are nearly white. Heterozygous dogs have the familiar merle combination of dilute and dark patches.

The interactions of alleles at a single locus are relatively easy to understand, but interactions of alleles and genotypes among different loci can be complicated. Some genotypes (specific combinations of alleles) at one locus can mask the expression of information at a second locus. This is somewhat like dominance and recessiveness but is an interaction of multiple loci instead of the interaction of alleles at only a single locus. In this situation the genotype causing the masking is referred to as epistatic, while the one that is masked is hypostatic.

Examples of epistasis come from coat color. The allele for black color in most dog breeds is dominant, and epistatic to the locus that causes colors such as sable or black and tan (Figure 2.6). The black color hides the combinations of black areas and tan areas typical of the colors produced by alleles at the other locus. A different locus hosts a recessive epistatic allele that results in yellow (or red) color that similarly hides the sable or black and tan patterns. The interaction of these loci can be complicated. One locus has a dominant allele that is epistatic to the second locus. The third locus has a recessive allele that is epistatic to that same second locus. The important concept is that certain genotypes at some loci mask the expression of the genotype of other loci.

Both dominance and epistasis function to hide a part of the genome. The masked information can be revealed by targeted breeding strategies and can also pop up as a surprise in a number of breeds following the mating of two animals that have identical masked information. Genetics is a fascinating way to attempt to unravel the hidden potential of animals. This can be done to produce desirable phenotypes, or to avoid producing undesirable phenotypes. Understanding that dominance and epistasis can mask portions of the

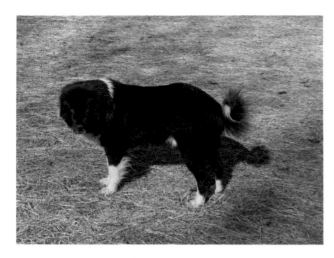

Figure 2.6 The allele that causes black color in most dog breeds is epistatic to other important loci that affect color. It hides the information at those loci. Photo by DPS.

genetic material is a huge step in understanding how to use genetics to achieve desired results by either unmasking genetic information, or by ensuring that it remains masked and unexpressed.

Breeders have a real advantage when dealing with traits that are governed by a single locus, or those traits where only a few loci are involved. The character of the alleles as discrete pieces of information means that they are relatively easy to follow through generations. In contrast, several important traits are controlled by many genes at many loci. Many conformational traits and behavioral traits fit into these polygenic control situations. Polygenic traits (hip dysplasia is a good example) are much more challenging for breeders, because many individual pieces of genetic information go into the final phenotype and are therefore difficult to tease out and individually identify and track from generation to generation.

Many people expect that genetics will be the key to ensuring specific outcomes for every mating decision. This can be true in some rare situations that involve minimal genetic variation but is an unrealistic expectation in most situations that involve real animals in real settings. It is generally more accurate to view genetics as constraining the possible outcomes of a mating to a relatively narrow range. While this outcome is broader than a single desired end point, it is still useful because it is narrower than the full range of outcomes that can occur when genetics is ignored. Narrowing the range of outcomes can be especially useful for breeders but is different than a guarantee that a breeder will achieve a final single desired goal each and every time.

2.2 *Gene Movement Through Generations*

Genetic material moves from generation to generation in a manner that is well characterized. At the most basic level each individual animal gets half of its genetic material from its sire, and half from its dam. In its own turn, each animal contributes half of its genetic material to each of its offspring. Each parent always contributes half of its genetic material to each of its offspring, but it is a somewhat randomly different half for each offspring.

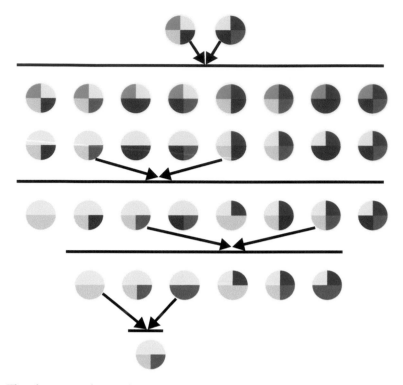

Figure 2.7 This diagram is for two loci and follows them through five generations. The colors represent distinct alleles within two loci. The "cool" locus on the top half of each individual has three alleles to begin with: light blue, medium blue, and dark blue. The "warm" locus on the bottom half also has three alleles: gold, dark brown, and maroon. The alleles can combine in various ways throughout the generations. In the second generation, all the alleles from the two original animals are present and the offspring can include any combination of these. Selecting two mates that lack the medium blue allele assures that it is missing in the third generation and cannot be regained. This results in fewer genotypes in that third generation. A similar fate occurs with the maroon allele as it fails to pass along to the fourth generation. Selection of breeding stock from that fourth generation has finally resulted in only a single genotype being produced in the fifth generation. The initial variation has been reduced drastically, even though along the way it has generated combinations of the alleles that were different from those in the original parents. Figure by DPS.

The pairing, halving, and renewed pairing of the genetic information at each generational step is possible because the information exists in a duplicated form related to the paired chromosomes. Imagining the juggling of genetic combinations at each generational step makes it possible to greatly increase the odds of producing outcomes that are desired by individual breeders (Figure 2.7).

The specific half of an animal's genome that is transmitted to its offspring is established by two main mechanisms:

- random segregation of chromosomes
- crossing over.

These both have important consequences for the way in which the genomes move through the generations.

Random segregation of chromosomes occurs because each parent can only transmit one chromosome from each of its pairs to its offspring. The offspring's pair comes as one from the dam and one from the sire. The result is that only half of the original information from a parent makes it to the specific individual offspring that is produced by the egg or sperm cell in question. However, dog reproduction produces litters that usually contain multiple puppies, so the fact that each pup receives one or the other of the chromosomes can lead to fairly broad sampling of the parental genetic material. Some puppies get one chromosome, while others get the alternative chromosome.

Crossing over further aids the mixing of genetic material from generation to generation (Figure 2.8). The paired chromosomes inside the progenitors of each egg and sperm cell have the opportunity to swap over varying lengths of their genetic information. This process occurs between the two chromosomes in each pair as they match up before splitting into the final egg or sperm cells. Crossing over involves the swapping over of one section of the maternal chromosome with the corresponding section of the paternal chromosome that is the same length. This mixes up the paternal and maternal contributions more evenly than could occur from the transmission of an entirely intact maternal or paternal chromosome. However, the mixing from crossing over is fairly limited. Crossovers usually occur at the rate of slightly over one crossover per chromosome per generation. That means that long stretches of both the maternal and paternal genetic information tend to remain intact from generation to generation. It also means that long strings of ancestral information are more likely to remain intact after a few generations than they are after many generations since

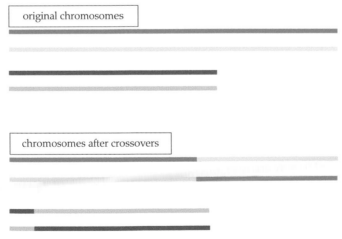

original chromosomes

chromosomes after crossovers

Figure 2.8 In the process of "crossing over" a chromosome exchanges lengths with its paired mate at each generational step. In this example, the "blue" chromosome has a crossover event about midway, which mixes the maternal and paternal contributions fairly fully. The "gold/dark brown" pair, in contrast, has a crossover that is towards one extreme end, so the mixing is less complete, and the parental information remains more intact. Over several generations the crossovers do tend to mix the original genetic material more fully, because they are fairly random in the specific sites at which they occur.

each generational step provides at least one more opportunity for mixing. Those opportunities obviously increase as the number of generations add up.

The constraint imposed on the genome by virtue of the organization of genetic loci along the length of a chromosome means that the mixing of alleles from generation to generation is fairly incomplete. Transmission across generations proceeds as chunks of either maternal or paternal information related to the position on an individual chromosome, the specific site of a crossover, and which chromosome makes it to the egg or sperm cell.

The movement of genetic information from generation to generation is constrained by these phenomena, and this determines how the genotypes of individual dogs are assembled from their parents. The sum total of genetic material in an entire population is also important, and also slightly different than considering individual dogs. The usual type of population involved in dog breeding is a single dog breed. Nearly all dog breeds are now "closed" in the sense that recruitment of the next generation is only from parents already registered in the breed. This means that no new genetic material can be introduced except fraudulently. It is important to maintain the genetic variations within a breed because once lost they are gone forever unless they can be brought back in from individuals outside the breed. The exception to the general recommendation to save all traits is those alleles that are responsible for disease, which need to be managed carefully because they are located adjacent to other pieces of genetic information. Some of those adjacent pieces might be particularly useful and could be lost along with the allele causing a problem unless breeders are very careful in how they manage genetic variation.

Some individual dogs within a breed have genetic variants that other members lack. This is important, because some variants, especially rare ones, are easily lost if breeders are not attentive to their presence and to procedures that can assure their retention. While some variation is likely trivial (color) or even deleterious (genetic diseases), much of it is neutral or even positive. Populations need variation to survive over prolonged generations. Managing variation effectively, while also preserving the uniformity that is a basic hallmark of dog breeds and their utility, is a huge challenge. Closed populations, especially dog breeds, need careful attention so that they maintain sufficient genetic variation to assure vitality and good vigor. This is an essential component of effective dog breeding and dog breed management if the goal is long-term and sustained success.

2.3 *Single Gene Inheritance*

The role of genetics is most often considered to be that of providing the background information that is needed to plan specific matings that will produce individual animals with desired specific traits. The way that genetics plays out in larger populations involves a broader scope and can be confusing. The details of the genetics of populations are important for dog breeders.

In general, transmission of single-gene traits is straightforward. These follow fairly simple rules, with the important recognition that random chance influences outcomes, and this is governed by certain peculiarities of statistics that are not always intuitive. Random effects, along with statistical phenomena, have a huge influence on whether the experience seen in a litter of puppies always agrees with the specific genetic theory involved in the control of the various traits of interest.

Most breeders will be familiar with the results of mating two carriers of a recessive gene. The ratio in the offspring is 25% homozygous dominant non-carriers, 50% heterozygous carriers (these first two classes have the same phenotype, despite their different genotype), and 25% homozygous recessives that express the recessive gene in their phenotype. This is the common 1:2:1 ratio of genotypes (Figure 2.9), but because two of those genotypes are phenotypically identical, the phenotypic ratio is 3:1 (Figure 2.10). The 3:1 ratio is achieved by adding two genotypes together (the homozygous dominant "1" and the heterozygous "2") because they are identical by phenotypic appearance.

Genetic ratios generally prove true in large populations. Small populations (such as single litters) frequently have fairly sizable deviations from these ratios. This is due to the chance involved in the transmission of the two alleles. Sometimes chance drives it one way, sometimes it drives it another way. Statistics describe the way that random events occur and assures that despite an average 50:50 split in the transmission of the alleles in large populations, some litters will have substantial deviations from the expected ratio. These deviations do not indicate that the science is incorrect. They only indicate that random chance can skew things one way or the other.

Chance is almost certain to skew the results in some individual litters, especially when large numbers of litters are involved. Statistical probability indicates that one allele of a heterozygote should be passed along 50% of the time, but in a very large number of matings very few litters will reflect either a 0% or 100% transmission rate. The rules are important, but it is equally important to remember that exceptions to them are certain to occur when a

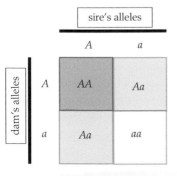

Figure 2.9 This is a "Punnett Square" that can help breeders to predict the results of a mating. In this case, both sire and dam are heterozygous *Aa*. If the sire's alleles are put across the top and the dam's along the side, then the various combinations can be put into the squares to which they contribute. Mating two heterozygotes gives a ratio of one homozygous dominant, two heterozygous, and two homozygous recessive. Figure by DPS.

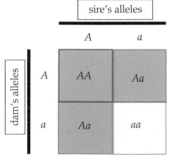

Figure 2.10 A 3:1 ratio comes from the fact that in many allelic interactions there is complete dominance. This makes the phenotype of the homozygous dominant and the heterozygous animals identical, adding them together into only a single phenotypic class. Figure by DPS.

large number of litters are considered. An example is the sex ratio within a litter of puppies. While the ratio of male and female puppies is right around 1:1, many individual litters deviate from this. Some litters, even large litters, have only male or only female puppies.

Despite deviations from the expected outcomes, an important detail is that single genes bring with them specific phenotypic ratios as they pass through the generations. These ratios are the hallmark of single genes at work and reflect how the two alleles interact. A few of these ratios are fundamental:

- The ratio 1:1 (or, more accurately, 2:2 to reflect the transmission of both alleles that each parent contributes) occurs following the mating of a heterozygous animal to a homozygous recessive animal. Half of the offspring are heterozygous for the recessive allele and do not express it, half express the recessive allele.
- The ratio 3:1 is the classic ratio for mating two carriers of a recessive gene. The "1" in this instance is the recessive phenotype, the "3" is the dominant phenotype.
- The ratio 1:2:1 is the classic ratio for mating two heterozygotes with either an incompletely dominant or codominant allele. In this case the three genotypes are accurately reflected in three phenotypes.
- The ratio 7:1 can be surprising but is fairly frequently encountered in situations where rare recessive mutations are present, new mutations have occurred, or a recessive allele is introduced into a population that previously lacked it. Recessive alleles do not express in the phenotype until homozygotes are produced, and they escape detection until this occurs. In situations where a recessive allele is rare, this most often happens after the mating of an initial heterozygote with its offspring (usually sire to daughters) or with its half-siblings. The first generation in this situation is a mating of the first heterozygote to homozygous dominant mates (Figure 2.11). The result is the expected 2:2 genotypic ratio with a 4:0 phenotypic ratio expressed due to the complete dominance. Half of the offspring are phenotypically normal homozygotes and half are phenotypically normal heterozygotes that carry the unexpressed recessive allele. When these two types of phenotypically normal offspring are mated back to the phenotypically normal heterozygous parent, the matings are of two sorts. Half of the matings are heterozygote to homozygote and no affected offspring are produced. The phenotypic ratio is 4:0. The other half of the matings are heterozygous carriers to one another. This yields the classic 3:1 ratio. The two sorts of matings cannot be distinguished phenotypically so the offspring are pooled together. Adding the 4:0 ratio to the 3:1 produces a 7:1 ratio.

Other ratios are possible, and generally indicate that something beyond the usual dominant and recessive situation is occurring. This includes multiple loci acting to produce a phenotype, and in that case the various ratios basically just get added together. This can become complicated when epistasis is involved (Figure 2.12).

An important deviation in ratios is reflected in a 2:1 ratio (Figure 2.13). This indicates that one of the genotypes is missing, usually because one of the homozygotes is not viable. All the other ratios are built on fours instead of threes. This makes perfect sense when it is remembered that the ratios are a consequence of paired information, so that they are built

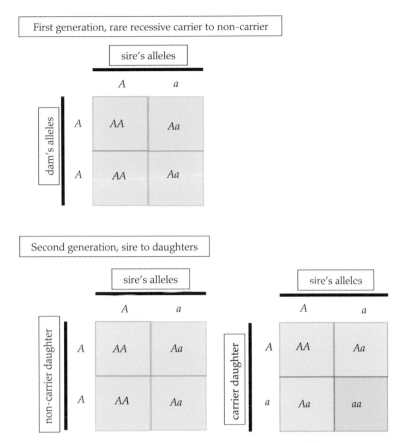

Figure 2.11 The 7:1 ratio usually arises when a carrier of a recessive allele mates to its own offspring. This can be a surprising ratio but is especially common with new mutations because they are initially so rare that two unrelated dogs are unlikely to both be carriers. Figure by DPS.

on powers of two. When one genotype is missing, something is causing loss. This is usually a loss during early development and the puppies with that specific genotype are simply not available to be counted at birth. Such alleles do result in smaller litters, but that detail is often overlooked by most breeders.

A mental picture that can help is to imagine individual alleles as different colors in a bowl full of mixed dry beans. Each individual allele (bean) retains its identity (color) and can be pulled out of the mix by careful planning. They never lose their individual identity; despite being mixed up in different combinations.

2.4 *Polygenic or Quantitative Inheritance*

Traits that are governed by many genes acting together do not follow these simple ratios. They are indeed genetically controlled, but the control is more complicated than the situations governed at a single locus. For these traits, the assessment is more a question of "how much" or "how many" than the simple "present or absent" that is true of most traits

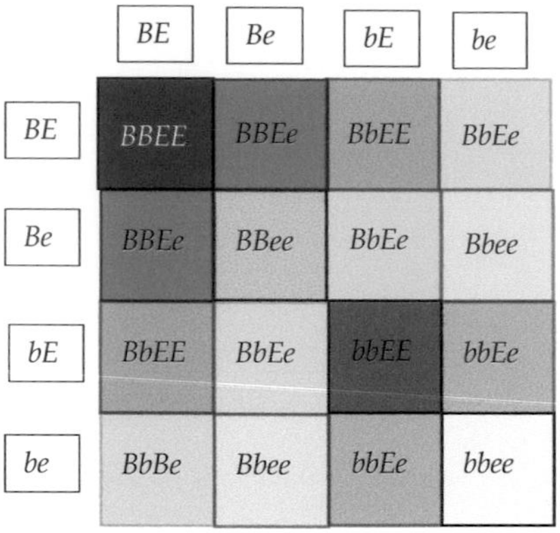

	BE	Be	bE	be
BE	BBEE	BBEe	BbEE	BbEe
Be	BBEe	BBee	BbEe	Bbee
bE	BbEE	BbEe	bbEE	bbEe
be	BbBe	Bbee	bbEe	bbee

Figure 2.12 Adding multiple loci together becomes complicated. If both parents are heterozygous at the same two loci, the genotypic ratio is 1:2:2:1:4:1:2:2:1. Each genotype in the figure is shaded distinctly. The phenotypic ratio can vary, depending on the mode of interaction by the alleles within a locus as well as whether there is any epistasis. With complete dominance at both loci, the ratio is 9:3:3:1. In this situation, all the "blue" individuals have identical phenotypes, as do the "tan" individuals, the "brown" individuals, and likewise, the double-recessive homozygote "pale" animal. Epistasis collapses these even further. Retriever color is controlled by black being dominant to chocolate (*B* and *b*), while yellow is a recessive genotype that is epistatic to both (*E* is nonyellow, *e* is yellow). This collapses the recessive genotypes (*ee*) into one phenotype, leading to a final 9:4:3 ratio of colors in the puppies, because the "tan" and the "pale" genotypes in the figure become indistinguishable. Figure by DPS.

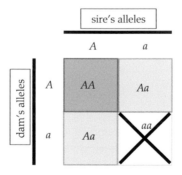

Figure 2.13 A 2:1 ratio usually indicates that one homozygote is nonviable and is therefore not present to be counted. Figure by DPS.

controlled by single genes. The "how much" traits controlled by multiple genes are called quantitative traits, in contrast to the "either/or" traits that are called qualitative traits and that tend to be governed by simpler genetic mechanisms. Rather than a mixture of individually identifiable dry beans, the polygenic quantitative traits are much more like mixing hot and cold water. The individual hot and cold contributions are nearly impossible to sort back out again.

Measurements of a quantitative trait generally fall along a bell-shaped curve, with few dogs at either extreme or most somewhere in the middle (Figure 2.14). Quantitative traits

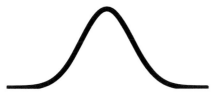

Figure 2.14 The bell-shaped curve is a common distribution for traits like height, weight, speed, and conformational traits. Most dogs in a population (a breed is a good example) fall in the middle of the range, with only a few that are at either extreme. Figure by DPS.

usually have multiple genes that affect them and have profound environmental contributions. Hip dysplasia is a good example, because the result in an individual dog is achieved by adding diet, management, exercise, and genetic potential. Great genes in a poor environment might have only a moderate outcome, while lousy genes in a great environment can actually do pretty well.

Quantitative traits are important, and include many conformational traits, speed, and other traits that vary continuously from a low point to a high point. A somewhat counterintuitive phenomenon is that the dogs at the extreme ends of a bell-shaped curve generally do not reproduce as extremely as their own phenotypes would suggest. This is for complicated reasons. At the more positive end, it is certain that the dog has good to excellent genes, but also that it had an optimal environment. That dog's puppies will get a hefty dose of decent genes, but their environments will vary, which will pull some puppies back toward the mean of the original bell-shaped curve. For this reason, only rarely does a truly extreme animal outproduce its own extreme phenotype.

An important subtype of quantitative, or polygenic, traits are those that have a threshold (Figure 2.15). The key concept here is that below a certain threshold of the number of genes, no expression of the trait is evident. Over that threshold the relative number of genes affecting the trait has an additive effect, with higher numbers leading to more extreme expression. Several structural cardiac defects are among these. Managing these traits is difficult. Dogs that are just below the threshold will not express the trait but can contribute sufficient alleles to their offspring (depending on their mate) so that their offspring can express the defect.

2.5 *Epigenetics*

Epigenetics is emerging as an important aspect of the overall function of the genome. The significance of epigenetics is still unfolding, and many details remain to be revealed.

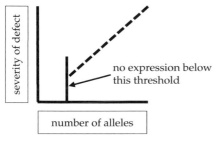

Figure 2.15 Polygenic threshold traits are especially challenging because normal animals can have several alleles that contribute to the trait, but without any expression. Figure by DPS.

The key concept is that expression and function of the specific sequences in the genetic code can be modified in various ways by a variety of biochemicals that are attached to the code itself. They do not change the code, but instead they modify how that code can be translated into a final product.

Many of the epigenetic effects are related to what can broadly be described as environmental influences. This can be a somewhat troubling principle. It can be taken to an extreme viewpoint that decrees that the environment is shaping the breed population as strongly (or even more strongly) than the underlying genetic code itself. The genetic code remains important, although these epigenetic influences do shape its final expression.

An important detail is that epigenetic influences can alter the expression of the genome for at least a few future generations. This affects breed management in a few ways. Two genetically identical dogs that experience quite different environments may well go on to pass along their genetic influence somewhat differently due to differences in the expression (not the presence!) of the various alleles in their own offspring. An example that some astute breeders have noticed in some lines is that the overall quality and ability of puppies produced late in a bitch's breeding life are somewhat below those produced during her prime years. This is likely due to epigenetic influences that accumulate as she ages.

It is difficult to make a broad recommendation on how to include epigenetics in selection decisions, other than to state that environments should ideally allow for candidate breeding dogs to fully express their genetic potential. This means appropriate nutritional support as well as attention to the physical condition of breeding stock so that fetuses get the best uterine environment possible. It is also important to note that an individual dog that is genetically important, but that is salvaged from a poor environment, may not produce up to its full potential.

2.6 Mating Strategies

Maintaining breeds as healthy and viable genetic resources should be the goal of each dog breeder and every association or registry involving dog breeders. This effort ideally involves different breeders using different breeding strategies. Each breeding strategy has different consequences for the individual kennel as well as for the breed. Each breeder must tailor a breeding strategy for the specific mix of philosophies, situations, and goals that are unique to the dogs that the individual breeder stewards. No single strategy fits all situations; there is no "single best answer." Instead, each strategy serves as a wise and appropriate choice for certain goals and systems. Having a variety of approaches, all within a single breed, works well for breed maintenance. The overarching goal is to assure a viable genetic structure for individual dogs and for the entire breed. This produces the best chance for the breed's long-term survival and productivity.

The mating strategies that breeders most commonly use include inbreeding, linebreeding, linecrossing, and outcrossing. Crossbreeding is another breeding strategy, and while breeders will object to including crossbreeding in a discussion of breed maintenance, including it helps to more fully flesh out what each of these strategies does to a population. The inclusion of crossbreeding in the discussion helps to explain some of the details of the other strategies that are more likely to be used in a dog breeding operation, even though it has no role in breeding purebred dogs.

Understanding how each of these strategies functions is important for breeders regardless of their personal goals. These terms all have slightly different definitions for separate groups of breeders, but the key fact is that the pairing of animals has varying outcomes depending on the degree of relationship of the specific dogs that are mated. The degree of relationship can be determined by evaluating pedigrees, or more directly by advanced DNA techniques. The pedigree of a candidate breeding dog is the first starting point. It is a record of an animal's ancestry, and all breeders should be able to read and understand a pedigree (Figure 2.16).

The results of each of the different breeding strategies are subjective points along a continuum that vary from completely inbred and uniform at one end to completely crossbred and widely variable at the other end (Figure 2.17). The exact point along this line at which the boundaries between inbreeding, linebreeding, linecrossing, and crossbreeding should be drawn is subjective. Despite that lack of tight definition, the effects of these strategies on populations are very real and need to be understood by conscientious breeders. Each strategy has a significant role in shaping animal populations, and for most breeds a combination of some or all of them is advisable for managing long-term success.

Individual animal	Parents	Grandparents	Great grandparents
dog	sire	paternal grandsire	paternal grandsire's sire
			paternal grandsire's dam
		paternal granddam	paternal granddam's sire
			paternal granddam's dam
	dam	maternal grandsire	maternal grandsire's sire
			maternal grandsire's dam
		maternal granddam	maternal granddam's sire
			maternal granddam's dam

Figure 2.16 A pedigree is a record of an animal's ancestry. Figure by DPS.

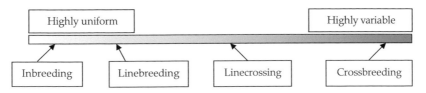

Figure 2.17 The various breeding strategies are points along a continuous line. Each is appropriate for specific goals and philosophies and is inappropriate for others. Figure by DPS.

From the outset, it is important to note that selection is the main factor that changes allele frequencies in a population. Nearly all dog breeders do indeed select their dogs, and selection is therefore a key component of breeding programs. Despite this, it remains important to understand that the different breeding strategies do not inherently change gene frequencies on their own. They only do this when they are coupled with selection. Selection changes allelic frequencies, which changes the genetic package of a breed. The breeding strategies can and do change the relative number of heterozygotes and homozygotes, which potentially exposes the genes to various levels of selection pressure. The final makeup of the population looks somewhat different depending on the breeding strategy. This is due to differences in the frequency of homozygotes and heterozygotes that are the result of the different strategies. However, the only way to deliberately change allele frequencies is through selection.

2.6.1 Linebreeding and Inbreeding

Linebreeding and inbreeding are only different from one another in degree. Both strategies involve the mating of related animals. One definition that separates these is "it is linebreeding if it works, and inbreeding if it doesn't work." This definition has some merit but does not serve as a very accurate guide for breeders as to the specifics of the two techniques.

Any mating of related dogs is technically inbreeding. The degree of relationship between any two dogs varies from distantly related to closely related. A practical definition that can help guide breeding practices sets the cut-off point for inbreeding as the mating of first-degree relatives. First-degree relatives include offspring, parents, and siblings (Figure 2.18). Although this is only one possible definition among many, it usefully separates inbreeding from linebreeding at a defined point. This definition works fairly well as a boundary between lower levels of related breeding that are generally tolerated quite well in all populations (linebreeding), and higher levels of related breeding that can hit barriers in many populations if not carefully monitored (inbreeding).

Linebreeding can be considered as the mating of related animals that have more distant relationships than first degree. Matings of aunt to nephew and grandparent to grand

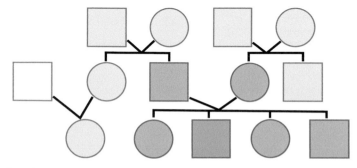

Figure 2.18 In this chart, males are squares, and females are circles. The dark blue individual is the one of interest. All the brown individuals are first degree relatives, which would classify a mating to the blue individual as inbreeding. The tan individuals are related, but more distantly, so mating any of them would be classified as linebreeding. The pale individual is unrelated, and so a mating would be classified as an outbreeding. Figure by DPS.

offspring could all be included here. Also included are more distant matings, such as between cousins.

Linebreeding and inbreeding both result in increased homozygosity, which means an increase in genetic uniformity of offspring. The genetic uniformity can be especially noticeable if these strategies are accompanied by appropriate selection practices. Linebreeding increases genetic uniformity because parents are related and therefore descend from a common and limited gene pool, which means that they have limited genetic variation to pass along to their offspring. Uniformity of appearance and performance of linebred dogs springs directly from this fact. The uniformity can be for anything, such as good looks, performance, or some other trait. Uniformity could also be for poor looks, performance, or some other trait. The initial animals, as well as selection practices, determine the relative quality of the product. In addition, the degree of relationship of the parents helps to influence the degree of uniformity in the offspring. The closer the relationship, the more uniform the offspring. And, if inbreeding is practiced over several sequential generations, the relationships become ever closer and uniformity increases.

An especially important historical note is that some level of linebreeding and inbreeding were the usual strategies for the establishment of breeds. These two breeding strategies can be coupled with selection to increase uniformity, and therefore predictability. These are the hallmarks of any breed. The very essence of a breed is that it has sufficient genetic uniformity for predictability. In that regard, both inbreeding and linebreeding can be effective in achieving the status of dog populations as true genetic breeds.

When linebreeding is coupled with selection (which it usually is), the result is a productive, predictable gene pool. Despite the very real advantage of this strategy, potential problems can occur in linebred populations. These problems are even more common in inbred groups. Common problems include loss of general vigor and especially loss of reproductive performance, characterized as both a decrease in conception rates and a decrease in litter sizes (Figure 2.19). In addition, inbred groups can have an increased rate of expression of undesirable recessive traits due to increased frequency of homozygotes. Skilled selection can help offset these potential drawbacks so that several linebred and inbred genetic resources (whether entire breeds or strains within breeds) are indeed productive, vigorous, and reproductively sound. The success of some linebred (or inbred) populations in no way eliminates the need for caution when breeders embark upon a strategy of inbreeding or linebreeding, because the risk of a negative outcome is very real and always needs to be considered.

A few breeds have shown great resistance to inbreeding, and these exceptions to the general rule are important. Unfortunately, they also can lull breeders into a false sense

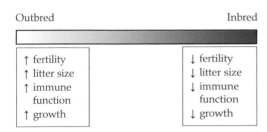

Outbred   Inbred

↑ fertility	↓ fertility
↑ litter size	↓ litter size
↑ immune function	↓ immune function
↑ growth	↓ growth

Figure 2.19 Inbreeding and outbreeding have opposite influences on populations, both of which can be used to good advantage by thoughtful breeders. Figure by DPS.

of security that inbreeding is of no threat to any line. Exceptions are interesting, but they are the successes that just happen to survive and therefore can be noticed while the failures are not around to gain that same notice. If twenty or so lines are started with intense inbreeding, only about two are likely to survive for several generations. The remainder will succumb to inbreeding depression and to eventual extinction if outcrosses are not used to reverse the effects of inbreeding. These effects include an increased rate of expression of fatal conditions along with a more general failure of reproductive success. Unfortunately, it is impossible to predict in advance which strains will survive inbreeding and which will succumb to it, even though some modern genetic testing modalities can help to make this prediction. Consequently, all strains, bloodlines, and breeds should be managed as if inbreeding depression is a real, if potential, threat.

Some kennels have practiced linebreeding or inbreeding as a successful strategy over several generations. In these situations, it is tempting for the breeders to ignore the very real risks of long-term inbreeding strategies because their own personal experience varies from the general rule. In multiple cases, the inbreeding that continued successfully for several generations suddenly hits a generation where vitality and reproduction fail precipitously. This is an important warning. Many populations reveal little sign that inbreeding is reaching unacceptable levels until it is too late! Many breeders firmly believe that their own breed or bloodline is completely resistant to inbreeding, only to find out that the next generation proves them wrong.

While several cautions have been raised against inbreeding and linebreeding, it is equally important to remember that these are extremely useful breeding strategies in some situations and can be used to achieve specific goals. The deleterious effects only usually surface after several sequential generations of linebred or inbred matings. Over shorter periods they can each serve positive roles in managing gene pools. Inbreeding and linebreeding are power tools that are effective when used appropriately, and dangerous when used carelessly.

2.6.2 *Outcrossing*

Outcrossing involves the mating of animals that are not related and is the philosophical and biological opposite of linebreeding. Outcrossing and outbreeding are synonyms, and the resulting offspring are commonly characterized as outbred, as contrasted to inbred. Outcrossing can be subdivided into two subgroups: crossbreeding and linecrossing. Crossbreeding is the mating of animals from two different breeds. Linecrossing is the mating of unrelated animals from within the same breed, and usually these matings occur between animals from two different bloodlines within the breed. This is the origin of the term "linecrossing." For many breeds, the extent to which animals truly have no relationship is debatable. The key concept here is the focus on "related" versus "unrelated," which will be explored further below.

Crossbreeding (mating dogs from two different breeds) is a fascinating phenomenon, partly because different results occur depending upon which generation is considered. The first stage is the initial cross. A breeding strategy that has become increasingly popular is the production of the modern varieties of "designer dogs" that are formed by an initial cross of two specific breeds, such as the Labradoodle that comes from mating a Poodle with a Labrador Retriever. More historic uses of the same strategy were commonly used to produce working dogs for specific situations such as the "lurchers" used for vermin control that were produced by mating sighthounds, herding breeds, and terriers in different combinations. Similarly, hounds for coursing coyotes were often crosses of Greyhounds with other sighthound breeds that were selected for being more aggressive hunters. The speed of the Greyhound, along with the hunting prowess of the Scottish Deerhound or Borzoi, produced useful and capable dogs that excelled at a specific task.

The initial cross of two breeds generally results in a very consistent product in the dogs of that first generation, known as the "F1" generation for "first filial" (Figure 2.20). However, when that initial generation is itself used for reproduction, the results start to become increasingly variable as the components get teased out into many new combinations. This variability is not all bad. When combined with selection, the excellent individuals can be skimmed off and used for their superior performance. The phenotypic excellence of the F1 dogs that result from crossing many different breeds can easily lull breeders into thinking that this strategy works over the long term for many generations. It can be a wonderfully productive strategy, but it only works for maximum benefits over the short-term (that F1 generation) and therefore requires a constant supply of purebreds to put into the initial cross that the system depends on.

It is important to keep in mind that dog breeds have been developed over long periods of time and for specific purposes. Selection has played an essential role in the predictability of a breed's looks and ability. These traits spring from a relatively constrained gene pool, and crossbreeding diminishes the uniformity (and predictability) of that pool when the crossbred dogs are used for reproduction.

An especially cautionary note comes from the group of livestock guardian dogs. The dogs from these breeds process information differently than other breed groups, and this is the key to their ability and usefulness. Much of this is related to a lack of predatory behavior. This uniqueness springs from their genotype. When livestock guardian dogs are crossbred within this group of breeds, the resulting puppies are often useful and capable livestock guardians. When crossbred to dogs from breeds outside this group, the resulting puppies can end up expressing certain components of predatory behavior well beyond what the

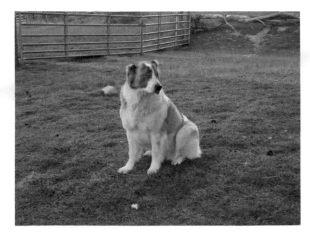

Figure 2.20 This successful livestock guardian is from a mating of two breeds from the same breed group: Central Asian Ovcharka and Maremma. She did her job successfully and well but was never used for reproduction. Photo by DPS.

parent from the non-livestock guardian breed normally has. In at least one instance, the product of a Kuvasz to Great Dane mating produced dogs that were hyper-predatory and would aggressively tear into horses.

A large, hyper-aggressive and predatory dog is a dangerous animal. The key to avoiding disasters such as this is to be keenly aware of the genetic background of the breeds in question, and to have specific goals in mind when crossing two breeds. The results of crossbreeding almost never have any constructive role in further breeding but can be quite useful in serving specific immediate needs. Crossbred dogs are a dead end for a breeder, even though some specific crossbred individuals may be wonderfully useful dogs.

Many of the disadvantages that arise from a linebreeding strategy (decreased vigor and reproductive efficiency) are enhanced under a crossbreeding strategy. Conversely, the advantages of using a linebreeding strategy (consistency and predictability) are diminished under a crossbreeding strategy. Each strategy therefore has a place in wise animal breeding systems, but they each serve vastly different goals. Purebred breeding, especially, needs to rely on approaches that support the closed gene pool of a breed over long periods of time.

Linecrossing is less extreme than crossbreeding because it occurs within a single breed. It has some of the same biological consequences as crossbreeding even though the crossing is contained within a single breed. This provides the benefits of crossbreeding without the loss of breed character and type. The variability in puppies produced by linecrossing is not as great as a cross between breeds, and the boost from hybrid vigor is not as great. Linecrossing can contribute to vigor, but it does moderately lower the predictably of production in following generations by virtue of creating animals that are more genetically mixed (heterozygous) than linebred animals are. Only a careful analysis of each individual situation will indicate whether this is a good tradeoff.

2.6.3 Defining Matings as "Related" or "Unrelated"

The exact point at which matings are classified as "related" (contributing to inbreeding), versus "unrelated" (not contributing to inbreeding) is impossible to define in absolute terms. Nearly all purebred matings are more closely related than matings to another breed are. This, after all, gets back to the whole point of breeds being genetic resources that spring from a single foundation and that have enough genetic uniformity to be predictable.

Two animals are unrelated if none of the ancestors of one occur in the pedigree of the other. As a useful general rule (with some important exceptions outlined below) the mating of any two animals that have no ancestors in common back to grandparents can be considered as outbreeding. The offspring will have no ancestors in common on either the sire's side or the dam's side back to the great-grandparents. Any relationship beyond this level is usually trivial and contributes so little to inbreeding that it is generally safe to ignore. At the other extreme, the mating of first-degree relatives (parent to offspring, full and half siblings) can be considered inbreeding because these animals are very closely related. Between these two extremes lies linebreeding, which varies in degree, but still lies at a level between severe inbreeding and outbreeding (Figure 2.21).

A warning that is important in many dog breeds is warranted. Some dog populations (whether bloodlines, individual kennels, or entire breeds) are linebred in consistent ways

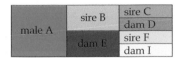

male A	sire B	sire C
		dam D
	dam E	sire F
		dam I

Mating to female E is inbreeding (son to mother)

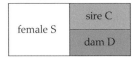

dam E	sire F	sire G
		dam H
	dam I	sire J
		dam K

Mating to female L is inbreeding (full brother to full sister)

female L	sire B	sire C
		dam D
	dam E	sire F
		dam I

Mating to female M is more distant inbreeding (half siblings)

female M	sire B	sire C
		dam D
	dam N	sire O
		dam P

Mating to female Q is linebreeding (cousins)

female Q	sire R	sire C
		dam D
	dam N	sire O
		dam P

Mating to female S is linebreeding (nephew to aunt)

female S	sire C
	dam D

Mating to female T is linebreeding (grandsire to granddaughter)

female T	sire U	sire A
		dam V
	dam N	sire O
		dam P

Mating to female W is an outbreeding (no relationship of mates)

female W	sire X	sire Y
		dam Z
	dam N	sire O
		dam P

Figure 2.21 Pedigrees of a male and several potential female mates demonstrating varying levels of inbreeding and linebreeding. Male A could be mated to each of these, and the common ancestors are color-coded to indicate the ancestors that are identical. Figure by DPS.

back to a few founders that were used to initially establish and expand the population. As the generations continue to develop, these early relationships can be so far back in the pedigree that breeders are unaware that two animals might indeed be fairly highly related. Some successful lines of dogs in some breeds are largely based on two successful founders, but this relationship might not be obvious unless extended pedigrees are examined. In some cases, dogs that are four or five generations removed from these founders are still up to 40% or even 50% of their genetic influence, even though that relationship may not be obvious in the parental and grandparental pedigree. Matings between two such dogs are indeed inbred despite having no ancestors in common back to grandparents (Figure 2.22).

The consequences of inbreeding that occurs in recent generations may be different from those that occurred in more distant generations. The devil is in the details. The blending of parental genetic material is governed by segregation of chromosomes, as well as by the crossovers at each generation that occur between the two members of a chromosome pair. The consequences of the crossovers compound over generations, so that the lengths of chromosomal fragments that remain intact are sequentially shortened (on average) as each generation is produced. The entire chromosome is still present, it is only that the original continuous lengths of the chromosome from distant ancestors becomes shorter and shorter, having been more thoroughly blended throughout the generations by the crossover

Kera KaraKitan

Parents	Grandparents	Great grandparents	
Baron Yape	Tanyo KaraKitan	Medun	Buyan KaraKitan
			Djesi
		Kusha KaraKitan	Kitan
			Gizda
	Bela	Arzan KaraKitan	Sharo Pepelonoviya
			Erma Karakitan
		Kalina II KaraKitan	Sharo Pepelonoviya
			Yantra KaraKitan
Kitana KaraKitan	Kysho	Kitan	Mager
			Yantra
		Duda	Sharo
			–
	Kysha	Chopar	Kitan
			Tundja
		Goldi	Churchil
			Yantra II .5.0

Figure 2.22 KaraKitan kennel used linebreeding very effectively to produce their reliable Karakachan livestock guardian dogs in Bulgaria. Relationships between animals from this bloodline can only be determined by examining extended pedigrees. This pedigree is complicated, and the several generations that are needed to fully convey the level of inbreeding will not fit on a single page. The ancestors with tan shading are all closely related, and the "yellow" ancestor is the result of a brother to sister mating. Despite the lack of overlap back to grandparents this is a heavily linebred pedigree, going back multiple ways to the ancestors of the "tan" animals. It is important to note that while "Bela" in the pedigree is linebred back to Sharo Pepelonoviya, the linebreeding to this animal then disappears because he no longer appears on both sire's and dam's sides of either Baron Yape or Kera KaraKitan. Figure by DPS.

events at each generational step. That makes the effect of inbreeding more consequential if it occurred in recent generations than if it occurred in the distant past because longer stretches of the chromosomes are more likely to be identical, and therefore homozygous.

Inbreeding is a real threat to viability, and while it can be managed, it should never be ignored. The consequences of the way in which dog breeds have traditionally been managed have resulted in an important long-term multigenerational experiment in just exactly what inbreeding can do to populations such as dog breeds. Inbreeding levels in dog breeds vary from breed to breed, and from breed group to breed group. Studies have shown a direct correlation between levels of inbreeding within a breed and enhanced levels of the incidence of diseases in general. Some of the consequences are direct manifestations of the deleterious alleles that all breeds have and that are likely to be paired up (and detrimental) following the mating of related dogs to one another. Other consequences are a bit more vague and are not related to specific alleles, but rather to the generally diminished level of genetic diversity in inbred populations. Consequently, inbreeding leads to declines in overall health and vigor. Inbreeding can be especially damaging to general canine health when it is coupled with selection for extreme expression of various traits.

These phenomena indicate that managing the level of inbreeding is extremely important for dog breeders if the goal is to have useful and healthy breeds in the future. Equally important to managing inbreeding is to assure that selection is occurring. In a few breeds, high levels of inbreeding seem to be tolerated very well, but these breeds are exceptions to an important general rule that inbreeding does cause depression. They are important exceptions to the general rule that inbreeding is best when carefully managed. There are situations where inbred matings make perfectly good sense, but caution is needed when this becomes a more general approach throughout a breed.

2.6.4 Linebreeding or Outcrossing: Which is Best?

The phenomena associated with linecrossing and linebreeding have different consequences, and each can be a logical choice for certain situations (Figure 2.23). These strategies each work well for specific philosophies and goals, and these vary from breeder to breeder. This is healthy for breeds. Philosophies might include conservation principles, performance utility, a high-profile program with name recognition, or others. Goals might include excellent temperament or a specific look or ability. These different philosophies and goals are all legitimate underpinnings for a breeding program. Specific goals and philosophies are important in driving decisions as to which strategy to use, and when to use it. The underlying philosophic question (why is the breeder breeding dogs in the first place?) is essential for all breeders but is not frequently asked. In the absence of a guiding philosophy and specific goals, breeding programs generally fail to make much progress. All breeders should develop a guiding philosophy, for this assures better progress and a more focused breeding program. Only then can the breeding strategies be used for maximum benefit.

Inbreeding tends to firmly and repeatedly establish traits in the offspring. Inbred offspring tend to be more consistent in reproducing their own type than are outbred individuals. Breeders can use this to their good advantage. However, breeders must keep in mind that prolonged multigenerational inbreeding will likely bring a decline in general vitality and reproductive fitness. The real risks of long-term inbreeding in no way limit the usefulness of short-term inbreeding that is targeted to accomplish specific selection goals within a bloodline or breed. Specific strengths and uses for inbred animals include using them for outcrossing to other lines to balance genetic founders within a breed, to increase vigor and vitality, or to reap the benefits by adding in some specific trait in a given line. Another wise use of inbreeding is to concentrate the genetic material of a superior animal so that the offspring can be used more broadly than is possible with a single dog.

Uniformity of progeny can be important for some breeding operations. Linebreeding is one strategy used to achieve this end in a purebred setting. Reasonably uniform animals that perform predictably are of great value. Obviously, the dogs of even the best breeding

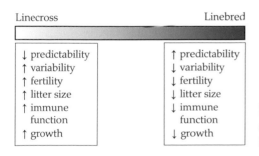

Linecross

↓ predictability
↑ variability
↑ fertility
↑ litter size
↑ immune function
↑ growth

Linebred

↑ predictability
↓ variability
↓ fertility
↓ litter size
↓ immune function
↓ growth

Figure 2.23 The benefits and risks of inbreeding and linecrossing tend to be opposite to one another. Figure by DPS.

programs are never going to be entirely uniform. The better performing ones will always be retained in favor of the lower performing ones. However, as the variation diminishes, the top and the bottom performers of the population approach one another, hopefully by the bottom coming up toward the top. This is indeed the impression received by viewing dogs from many long-term and successful purebred operations.

Linebreeding takes time and commitment. In contrast, linecrossing and crossbreeding can be quick fixes and are tempting strategies for a variety of reasons. One outcome of crossbreeding is initially phenomenal results, especially if the parents that are recruited for the crossbreeding are thoughtfully selected for complementary strengths. The boost of linecrossing is similar and comes from hybrid vigor. The downside of crossbreeding is the loss of a breed-specific genetic package that can then not be regained.

In contrast to crossbreeding and linecrossing, many older, high-reputation breeders of most breeds have used a linebreeding strategy that is coupled with selection to produce the animals and breeds that are highly desired by breeders today. For most breeds, too few breeders have long-term commitments. This is especially true for linebreeding and the development of consistent, productive lines that are predictable for performance.

Linebreeding and linecrossing can both be used to achieve good results within a single kennel when these strategies are alternated from generation to generation (Figure 2.24). This is accomplished by ensuring that linecross animals, rather than being further line-crossed, are preferentially linebred (backcrossed) to one of the specific lines that is in their own ancestry. Mating linecrossed animals back to one of their parental lines accomplishes this. That sort of mating then produces linebred animals once again, which can then be used in linecrossing. This strategy avoids multi-generation linebreeding with its attendant risks. While the resulting population will not be intensely linebred, some portions of the

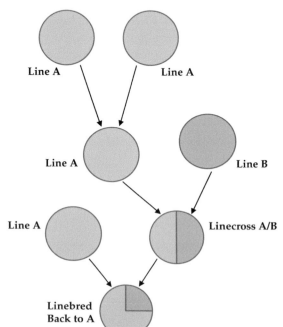

Figure 2.24 The effects of alternating linecrossing with linebreeding generation to generation. The proportion of genetic material from the different lines in each generation is indicated by the different proportions of each color. Figure by DPS.

overall population will indeed be moderately linebred. The linebred portion will have the benefits of linebreeding, but without much risk of the drawbacks that can possibly plague more long-term, multigenerational linebreeding programs. A breeding program that accomplishes the alternation of these strategies needs to be carefully planned and executed, and the results will usually reap great benefits for both the breeder and the breed.

A breed population is best served if multiple breeders are using slightly different breeding strategies, philosophies, and methods. The genetic health of a breed benefits if some breeders are linebreeding and others are linecrossing. This allows for successful genetic combinations to be developed in a variety of locations and conditions. This is good for both breeds and breeders. A single program and philosophy will not fit all situations, and breeders need to encourage diverse approaches and techniques. This requires coordination and cooperation among purebred breeders. Overseeing and facilitating this is an important role for breed associations but is often a role that is lacking.

2.7 Key Points

- Genes flow from generation to generation in specific ways that are based on the paired character of the genetic information.
- Genetic management is important, but it almost never achieves 100% predictability of a specific outcome.
- Genetic mechanisms determine best practices for managing traits.
- Single genes that interact in set ways are routinely easy to manage.
- Traits under control of multiple genes are more difficult to manage.
- Some traits have a threshold of expression that makes their management especially difficult.
- Selection changes gene frequencies and is the key to achieving desired outcomes.
- Inbreeding and linebreeding make a population more uniform and predictable.
- Linecrossing and outcrossing result in more genetic diversity and greater vigor.
- Most dog breeds should use both linebreeding and linecrossing to achieve the strengths of both while diminishing the drawbacks of both.

CHAPTER 3

Dog Evaluation

Evaluation is an important step in the selection of dogs for reproduction, and many different aspects should be considered. Evaluation and management of a young dog starts on day one out of the womb. Good breeders spend many, many hours socializing dogs, evaluating their structure, and assessing their temperament. There is no substitute for the time that the breeder spends on the evaluation process. Methods for evaluation vary greatly from trait to trait. Many traits are relatively easy to evaluate, others are notoriously difficult. The potential trap is that the traits that are easiest to evaluate will end up driving all decisions, to the exclusion of important aspects that are more difficult to evaluate (Figure 3.1).

Among those traits that have become easy targets for selection are an ever-expanding list of specific alleles for which there are genetic tests. Conformation is a somewhat more difficult target but can still be evaluated in a reasonably objective manner. Other characteristics, such as temperament and physical soundness, are much more difficult to evaluate, but are no less important for the long-term welfare and function of dogs. Many breeds have specific traits (physical or behavioral) that are related to the specific function of the breed. Evaluations for these can be difficult to acquire, and some are especially challenging if they are to be done by someone other than the owner or handler. Evaluations for these traits can quickly become subjective, which makes them more difficult but no less important.

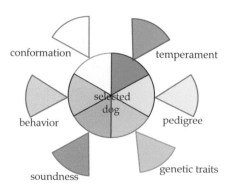

Figure 3.1 Many different aspects of a candidate dog influence the final decision on that individual's role in a breeding program. Figure by DPS.

Individual dogs are most often evaluated for their own single genes, functional ability, conformation, and temperament. A more nebulous factor is how the specific individual dog fits into the breed's population structure. This requires an understanding of the dog's breed structure and how various lines are related. Uncovering this is important, but it is unfortunately quite challenging in most situations.

The mechanics of evaluation are important, because the method by which traits are evaluated influences the validity and usefulness of the results. Methods of evaluation vary from objective genetic tests to the more subjective assessments of ability, working style, and position in a breed's population structure such as representing a rare bloodline. A broad range of individual and breed-related factors should all be considered when evaluating a candidate dog for reproduction.

The portion of dog breeding that is influenced by assessment must interact successfully with important details of the biology of dog reproduction. An inherent drawback in dog breeding is that canine reproduction cannot be postponed indefinitely. In an ideal situation it would be possible to limit reproduction to mature or even elderly dogs after they had proven their strength and utility over several years. Due to a host of biological peculiarities of dogs, this is rarely advisable because many dogs (especially bitches) will be unable to reproduce well if kept barren for several years running. The result of the biological influences is that a great deal of evaluation of candidate dogs needs to be based on predictions of performance and longevity rather than from actual measurements as the years progress. This is an important concept, because the final result depends on how accurately the predictive measurements do their job. Every step away from the actual genotype for a trait of interest introduces less and less accuracy into the final evaluation. This affects the overall utility of the various evaluations in making final selection decisions. Despite the limitations of predictive approaches, they must be used for many traits because no practical alternative is available.

Fortunately, a wide variety of modern tools and assessments are available to help breeders make wise decisions. Alongside these tools lie some more traditional methods that can tend to be overlooked as breeders opt for more modern and technological approaches. Traditional approaches do still have important uses today, and breeders ignore those at their peril.

Most successful animal breeders have a "good eye," which refers to a fairly intuitive sense that recognizes superior animals, as well as their potential to pass along that excellence to their offspring. These breeders know, almost instinctively, which matings will work and which will be less successful. This is a very subjective sense and can seem to be at variance with the more quantitative and statistical approach that has been followed by many animal breeders over the last several decades. One component of "eye" is a certain degree of critical assessment that notes any weaknesses along with any strengths.

It is important to remember that the traditional and the more modern approaches both have merit when selecting animals for reproduction (Figure 3.2). Combining them can greatly strengthen a breeding program. Unfortunately, the "eye of the master breeder" is currently likely to be discounted by many breeders. It is important to remember that this very traditional approach has been the one that originally produced the breeds that are enjoyed and valued today. Previous traditional approaches have produced excellence both

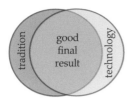

Figure 3.2 Combining traditional approaches with today's technology is more powerful than using either one alone. Figure by DPS.

in performance and in eye appeal and continue to do so. This is especially true when they are combined with the more modern or technological approaches.

Dogs that are intended for breeding, or that may be considered for a breeding program, should receive all the health testing recommended for their specific breed. Nearly all breed clubs have a health committee. Many breed clubs outline common genetic and congenital problems that affect the breed. This information is usually published either in the bylaws or on the breed club's own website. Health committees of breed clubs are the most up-to-date resource a breeder can use. The goal of these committees is to ensure, to the best of the club's and breeders' ability, that dog health and dog quality are becoming better with each generation.

Breeders need to pay special attention to the frequency with which some tests need to occur, as well as to the specific type of test required. It is important to remember the differences between phenotypic and genotypic health tests. Phenotypic results are prone to be influenced by genetics, nutrition, and environmental factors. This puts them a step away from the true breeding value of a dog, but for many traits this is as close as the evaluation can come. Genotypic tests rest on the DNA, so they more accurately reflect the animal's breeding value. Results of genotypic tests cannot be influenced by anything other than that individual's parental genetic make-up, which has already been established at conception.

Regardless of the specific approach they use, breeders shape their bloodline and their breed by the selection decisions they make. Decisions are based on a whole host of different factors, each of which brings potential strengths or weaknesses. The usual types of information people use when evaluating breeding animals include pedigree, performance records, ability, conformational analysis, and results from DNA tests. Understanding how these types of information can work together can help breeders to use the strengths of each one, while also avoiding the pitfalls that each of them can have when they are misused.

3.1 *Pedigree Evaluation*

Most dog breeders put great importance on pedigrees. A pedigree is an account of the ancestry of an animal and identifies specific individuals as sire, dam, grandsire, granddam, and so on (Figure 3.3). Pedigrees link an individual animal to specific ancestors and are of great value in establishing the relationships of animals within a breed so that inbreeding can be monitored. Pedigree analysis is a useful first step when choosing mates to produce the next generation.

Pedigrees do have the limitation of only offering a broad estimate of the genetic contributions of the ancestors. This is because the influence of ancestors in a pedigree is based on averages, which introduces some subtle and potentially confusing aspects. All animals

Individual animal	Parents	Grandparents	Great grandparents
individual dog	sire	paternal grandsire	paternal grandsire's sire
			paternal grandsire's dam
		paternal granddam	paternal granddam's sire
			paternal granddam's dam
	dam	maternal grandsire	maternal grandsire's sire
			maternal grandsire's dam
		maternal granddam	maternal granddam's sire
			maternal granddam's dam

Figure 3.3 Pedigrees are records of ancestry. Learning how to read them is an important skill for breeders. Pedigrees track the potential influence of ancestors on the current generation. Figure by DPS.

receive 50% of their genetic material from their dam and 50% from their sire, so the influences from the immediately previous generation are firmly set.

For generations further back than parents, though, the proportions of the influences from the ancestors in a specific ancestral generation can be much less certain. The 50% of the genetic material from a dog's sire (or dam) does not need to be made up from exactly 25% from that animal's sire and 25% from that animal's dam. This is due to the random segregation of the individual chromosomes within each pair and is also due to the specific site of any crossovers between the maternal and paternal chromosomes. While a relatively even contribution will be true on average, the exact proportion of the influence from each grandparent can vary considerably from one individual grand-offspring to another. This is one reason littermates vary from one another. This uneven representation back beyond parents contributes to the fact that some littermates are better candidates for reproduction than others, despite having identical pedigrees.

The result of all these details of the transmission of genetic material is that an exactly even contribution from ancestors back beyond parents is actually fairly rare, despite the fact that each parent must indeed contribute an even 50%. Within each pair of grandparents (maternal or paternal) it is common to have a disproportionately low or high contribution, made up by a correspondingly high or low contribution of the other grandparent of that maternal or paternal pair. The final total contribution from each of those pairs does end up being 50%, but the contribution of each of them to make up that 50% often varies (Figure 3.4).

This may seem to be a trivial detail, but the uneven contribution of distant ancestors is nearly certain to occur to at least some extent at each generation, and this varies among individual puppies that are full siblings. These uneven contributions become compounded over the generations. Once the contributions are uneven, the succeeding generations can never attain more than whatever contribution has been made by the previous generation.

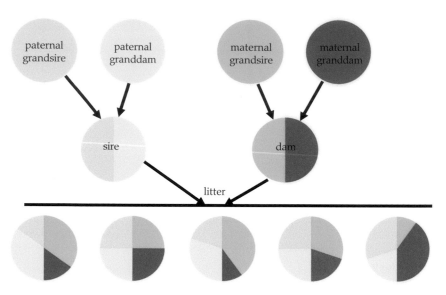

Figure 3.4 While the contribution of sire and dam to the next generation is always 50% each, the contributions of ancestors further back can be very uneven across members of a litter. Figure by DPS.

Basically, once the contribution from a specific ancestor is skewed one way or the other, it remains so down through the generations and becomes difficult, or impossible, to change it. This is true whether the contribution is an over-representation or an under-representation.

Pedigrees alone cannot accurately capture the phenomenon of unequal contributions of distant ancestors because pedigrees rest on the assumption that the members of each ancestral generation have contributed equally from generation to generation. This is correct on average and across large groups of dogs but is likely to be incorrect for nearly all animals if they are considered individually.

Despite this practical limitation, pedigrees are still incredibly useful as a first step in understanding relationships and should therefore never be overlooked. Their easy availability and relatively low cost make pedigrees a logical first step in evaluating the potential of a dog to make a positive contribution to a breeding program. This step can now be augmented by detailed DNA analysis, which adds important detailed information to the initial pedigree evaluation.

Pedigree evaluation can be done by evaluating the specific ancestors that are behind a dog, and how those ancestors are arranged in the pedigree. For example, if the same male is the sire of the individual's own sire and dam, then that individual dog is tightly inbred. This knowledge can affect how that dog's mates are chosen. The generation within the pedigree that warrants close examination will vary from situation to situation. In most cases the influence of an ancestor back beyond grandparents becomes relatively minor, with the important exception that in situations with considerable linebreeding or inbreeding even distant ancestors can become extremely important (Figure 3.5). One constructive use of pedigrees is to evaluate them for ancestors with an excellent and unique phenotype (conformation,

Pedigree for Pirin KaraKitan			
Parents	Grandparents	Great grandparents	
Sharo KaraKitan Roshaviya	Kysho	Kitan	Mager
			Yantra
		Duda	Sharo
			–
	Meda KaraKitan	Medun	Buyan KaraKitan
			Jessy
		Kusha KaraKitan	Kitan
			Gizda
Kitana KaraKitan	Kysho	Kitan	Mager
			Yantra
		Duda	Sharo
			–
	Kysha	Chopar	Kitan
			Tundja
		Goldi	Churchil
			Yantra II

Figure 3.5 This pedigree reveals inbreeding to the sire of both the sire and the dam. In addition, there is further duplication of the ancestors "Kitan" and "Yantra" because they also appear in the ancestry of the dams of both sire and dam. Some of this information "falls off" to the right because Buyan KaraKitan is a son of Kitan and Gizda, and Yantra II is a daughter of Yantra, the dam of Kitan. This pedigree resulted in a good, strong dog, but it remains important to know the details of the extended pedigree for a tightly linebred dog such as this. Figure by DPS.

performance, or other). Such dogs are good candidates for a linebred mating back to that excellent individual to maximize the chances of recapturing that dog's strength.

The evaluation of pedigrees can become arduous when many dogs are involved, but the astute breeder will know the individual excellent animals of the breed and will be able to recognize their names in a pedigree. Pedigrees are very useful in identifying relatively rare genetic influences that have in fact turned out to be excellent. It is especially important that these are not lost within a breed. Pedigree analysis can help to guide breeding and selection decisions by noting those excellent individuals.

Assessing a pedigree can determine if a candidate breeding dog comes from very common bloodlines or from bloodlines that are rarer. This detail can be very useful in guiding other assessments. In the case of a dog with very popular ancestors, the rigor of other evaluations must be at a high level. There is no sense in using a poor or average dog from popular bloodlines because so many other dogs are available to make that genetic contribution. In contrast, a sound but unexceptional dog with rare bloodlines might actually have a great deal to offer because such a dog can balance out the other more popular influences in a breed while at the same time not posing much of a risk that quality will be lost. Essentially, a dog from common bloodlines must be excellent to warrant broad use. A dog from rare bloodlines can be allowed more leeway, because much of what such a dog offers a breed is hidden from view in the genome.

3.1.1 Coefficient of Inbreeding

One way to capture the degree of linebreeding or inbreeding in a pedigree is the coefficient of inbreeding (COI). This number reflects the degree of relatedness between the dog's sire and dam. The COI specifically provides a measure of the probability that an individual dog is homozygous at a given locus, and that both alleles have originated from a single allele in a single ancestor. Although this is the specific basis for the calculations, the COI also predicts the overall degree of homozygosity at all loci in an animal due to the alleles having originated in an ancestor that appears on both the dam's side and the sire's side.

The values of the COI vary from 0, in a completely outbred dog whose sire and dam had no relationship, up to a theoretical maximum of 1 (Figure 3.6). A COI value of 1 would represent a dog that is completely homozygous due to ancestral relationships. For a host of reasons this is not possible, so it is wise to focus on the more practical range over which the COI varies in real populations. A few specific values help to put COI levels in perspective. COI values of 0.25 are produced by a parent-to-offspring mating, or by a full brother to full sister mating. This is a relatively high coefficient, despite the theoretical maximum going all the way to 1. In a practical sense these two types of mating are about as closely related as a mating can be, and therefore a COI of 0.25 is at the upper end of what is practically possible within a single generation. A higher COI is possible but requires close inbreeding over multiple generations in order for these relationships to add up throughout the pedigree.

The COI can be calculated by hand, but this is complicated and arduous to do in complicated pedigrees that have multiple repeats of several different ancestors. Dog pedigrees are especially likely to have multiple common ancestors in multiple ancestral generations. Most registries now do this calculation automatically and make the result known, often by putting it on the registration certificate. The COI is a useful guide to the likely degree of homozygosity in an animal. The higher the COI value, the more inbred the animal is, and the greater degree of homozygosity. An important detail is that the COI is not an indication of the quality of a dog, but it is an indication of the relative risk of inbreeding depression.

The COI is computed from the pedigree, and this involves comparing animal identities back several generations. The number of generations can be specified, and the resulting COI may well be different when considering the ancestry back to different generations. This generally presents no practical problem, and a COI that is calculated back to five or so generations is usually adequate. Going back further, for example to ten generations, rarely adds much more information, with the important exception being that this level of analysis may well be important and helpful in populations that have had a long history of linebreeding. Recent generations in this situation can miss the overall level of inbreeding, which in some examples can be quite substantial.

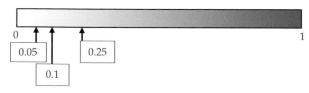

Figure 3.6 While inbreeding coefficients can theoretically run from 0 to 1, a coefficient of 0.25 is actually quite high. Populations generally aim for averages below 0.05, with a general recommendation that individual animals be below 0.1. Much higher coefficients do have strategic uses, as long as outcrosses are available to reduce the coefficient in the next generation. Figure by DPS.

The COI can be used in several ways, some of which are more constructive than others. General recommendations often suggest that the COI be kept below 0.10, or ideally at or below 0.05. These are good general rules when applied across an entire population, but important exceptions to this rule do arise when considering individual animals. Deviations from the rule are occasionally useful and wise in dog breeding. A dog with a very high COI might indeed be beneficial to a breeding program in some targeted instances, with the important warning that high levels of COI that occur over sequential generations are especially likely to lead to problems.

The COI does have a significant disadvantage based on the assumption of average allele transmission. In real life this may or may not occur, and likely fails to in most situations. The calculation of the COI assumes that alleles make it down through the generations in a statistically random fashion. The COI therefore accurately reflects the average situation across many animals but can never fully accurately catch the details for any given individual. The important detail is that if an allele fails to make it to a given generation, it can likewise not be available for any future generations in that lineage. Despite this drawback, the COI is a very useful measurement of the expected level of homozygosity in a dog.

A concept related to the COI is "kinship," which is a measurement of how closely two individuals are related to one another. Kinship is the COI that would result from mating two animals together, so it runs over the same range of values as COI and has the same host of factors that affect it. It can be calculated for theoretical matings before they are made or can be calculated for an individual dog and several mates as a sort of average. For example, a breeder with several females who may want to introduce a male into the kennel, is able to calculate his kinship with each bitch, as well as his average kinship to all of them.

In many situations a pedigree analysis can be coupled with thorough DNA testing to provide for a more accurate assessment of the actual level of homozygosity that has arisen from inbreeding. This will be explained in more detail below. DNA analysis is especially useful when close inbreeding is occurring, because carefully analyzed DNA results are the most accurate way to ascertain the real extent of genetic overlap between mates. This level of detail is usually not necessary when outbred matings are planned.

3.9 Evaluation of Phenotype: Structure and Other Traits

Phenotypic tests reveal important details about the quality of dogs that are candidates for reproduction. The information derived from a phenotypic test is fundamentally different than the information gleaned from genotypic tests, so each basic category needs to be understood to use them to their best advantage.

Phenotypic tests are especially useful in two basic sorts of situations. One is for diseases that are polygenic. A second is for those diseases that do indeed have simpler genetic mechanisms but for which the causative mutation has not yet been identified. Phenotypic tests are not directly predictive of the genotype, especially for polygenic diseases. As an example, a bitch with excellent hips as certified by the Orthopedic Foundation for Animals (OFA) will not always produce OFA Excellent rated puppies, but she has a better chance of producing phenotypically normal puppies than a bitch with radiographic evidence of hip dysplasia.

Phenotypic tests can have another disadvantage when compared to genotypic tests, due to limitations imposed by age of onset for many of the diseases. Phenotypic tests are only accurate once the disease has had sufficient time to manifest. Some tests, such as the OFA hip analysis, have a well-defined cut-off age. Other tests, such as those for certain eye or thyroid diseases, may need to be repeated throughout a dog's life because some of these diseases have a late and variable onset. For example, cardiac examinations may be recommended as a one-time event for some specific congenital abnormalities, while they might need to be repeated annually for certain diseases with a later onset. The specific recommendations depend on the predisposition to each disease for each breed. Many of the phenotypic tests have a requirement that they be performed by a board-certified veterinary specialist. A significant disadvantage of phenotypic tests for late-onset diseases is that it is possible for a dog to develop abnormal test results after it has already produced puppies. This is the reason that continued testing of breeding animals is essential for some diseases, even after the breeding retirement of the animal. This level of investigation is needed to track these diseases accurately through the lifespan of the dog, as well as to give an accurate indication of any risk to its descendants.

Structural evaluations are among the phenotypic evaluations that are important in assessing dogs for their relative strengths and weaknesses in a breeding program. Some structural evaluations are fairly objective, others are fairly subjective. Both types can play useful roles in the assessment of dogs.

Evaluating the hips of breeding dogs for hip dysplasia is one of the conformational evaluations with a long history, and the details can help to illustrate several important aspects that surround phenotypic testing for polygenic diseases. The OFA has certified the hip structure of dogs for many years. OFA evaluation is based on radiographic changes and requires that dogs be at least two years old when evaluated. A more recent procedure for hip evaluation is the PennHip procedure, which is based directly on the laxity of the hip joint and not on the degenerative changes that result from hip laxity. The PennHip procedure is more objective and can be accomplished as early as 16 weeks of age.

Hip dysplasia is a complicated trait, and the final clinical significance of it has powerful influences from genetics, environment, and the inherent sensitivity of the individual dog to react to pain (Figure 3.7). Breeders need to focus on the end goal of sound dogs, which is the result of all of the complicated factors added together. How best to achieve that goal is complicated. Evaluations that are based on the genetic mechanisms behind hip structure would be the most useful to achieve this goal but are currently unavailable, and it is unrealistic to think that they ever will be. Evaluations of phenotype that get as close to the genotype as possible are the next best option. The closer to the base of the cascade of events leading to final clinical unsoundness, the better. Assessments that measure characteristics that are further away from the basal components are less powerful in attaining final goals. This is why a direct and detailed evaluation of hip structure is much more accurate than measuring lameness or soundness, because those two traits have contributions from multiple contributing factors.

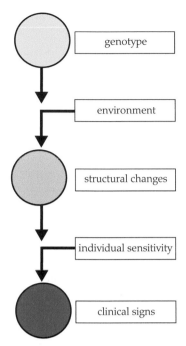

genotype

environment

structural changes

individual sensitivity

clinical signs

Figure 3.7 Disease from hip dysplasia is the result of several factors that all interact. Figure by DPS.

Other tests based on conformation or phenotype include evaluations of elbow conformation for developmental problems. These mirror the evaluations for hips but are generally more of a "yes/no" assessment of appropriate development of the bones, instead of the "how lax" assessment for hips.

Other certifications that are based on physical examination include several eye conditions and heart conditions. These are important in identifying dogs that express various diseases in these organs. An increasing number of diseases that affect these and other organs now have DNA tests available, which can greatly help breeders as they wisely and effectively manage them in their dog breeds. Test results are valuable pieces of information to help guide breeders to good breeding decisions, although they should always be put into the context of the entire breed and kennel. DNA tests are especially valuable for diseases with an onset late in life, because they allow the wise mating of dogs younger than is possible when it is necessary to wait for the age of onset for the disease.

Certifications and assessments gain increased validity when they are objective rather than subjective. For some phenotypic traits it can be difficult to come up with appropriate methods for accomplishing a reasonable degree of objectivity. The assessment scheme for "brachycephalic obstructive airway syndrome" serves as a useful model in how to construct such an evaluation. In the USA, this system is managed by the OFA. A candidate dog's ability to breathe easily is evaluated and scored before moderate exercise and then again after moderate exercise. The key to the repeatability and objectivity of the assessment is that the scoring system is well described, and those doing the certification are specifically trained in performing and scoring the evaluation. This has allowed breeders in the United Kingdom and in America to use this tool in their quest to produce brachycephalic dogs that can breathe well during rest, work, and play.

Many of the evaluations of structural phenotype are geared to performance and not to superficial physical characteristics such as coat or color. The specific evaluations can vary widely depending on the breed involved, and include bench and ring shows, field trials, and other ways to assess a dog and its conformation and ability. Many of these evaluations are competitive, with the specific goal of ranking a group of dogs as to the relative ability or appearance of each one. The competitive aspect of this sort of evaluation often brings with it the very negative consequence of selecting animals for extreme phenotypes. At the heart of competition is the idea that one dog is better than another, or indeed that one dog is better than all of the others! While this may be true from a broad view, it also remains true that a balanced dog often serves its important role as a human companion or work partner much better than can an extreme dog. "Balance" is an important concept, that always needs to be kept in mind, and is notoriously difficult to recognize.

Selecting extremes of structural conformation can be hazardous because extreme phenotypes can come from genetic mechanisms that can easily be tipped over to unsoundness. Specific examples are likely to offend various readers, and any one person's specific list is likely to include things that others would think are perfectly acceptable. Breeds selected for very short faces do encounter multiple problems, as do those selected for small eyes. Extremes of slope of various conformational features can bring in attendant problems. These can be very difficult or impossible to correct in succeeding generations if the selection has removed the genetic variation leading to more balanced and sound types.

An example unrelated to dogs comes from sheep. A century ago, breeders of fine-wooled Merino sheep pursued heavily wrinkled skin as a strategy for increasing skin area and therefore wool production. That turned out to not be the case, and introduced other problems associated with wrinkles. The next century has involved great efforts in trying to remove the wrinkles, but the wrinkles that were fairly easy to put onto the sheep have proven very resistant to removal!

One strategy for avoiding the pitfalls of selecting for extremes or overuse of a single winning animal has been adopted by some livestock and poultry breeds. This procedure is called "card grading." It is unlikely to be adopted by dog breed clubs but does offer an interesting alternative to more usual forms of dog evaluation. Card grading involves a panel of three judges evaluating each animal independently for adherence to the breed standard (Figure 3.8). Animals are then classed as "superior breeding stock," "good breeding stock," "acceptable breeding stock," and "unacceptable for breeding." This sort of procedure is unlikely to completely replace the traditional showing of dogs with a single grand champion but does have several advantages that are now being incorporated into some competitions.

Card grading tends to remove the idea that one single animal is best and replaces it with a more balanced conclusion that multiple animals can each play different roles in producing the next generation. It also sends the signal that all dogs over a certain threshold of quality are useful in breeding programs. Card grading can be especially powerful in educating breeders when it is coupled with an explanation of reasons for the placing of the animals. One of the key benefits of card grading is that it recognizes that not all superior breeding animals have the same strengths. Equally important is the fact that not all dogs that are down in the "acceptable" range have the same potential for use in a breeding program. Some of these dogs will be excellent across the board except for a single flaw. They can

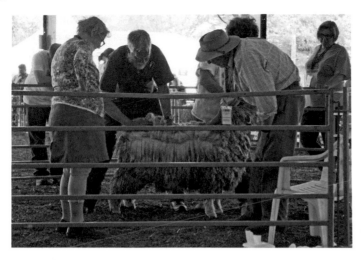

Figure 3.8 Card grading has proven quite useful to breeders of several livestock breeds. Photo by Alison Martin.

be mated wisely to correct that single flaw and may then be able to contribute their many excellent traits to the breed. In contrast, some dogs down in the "acceptable" range get there by having several different traits that lack excellence. Those dogs have much less to offer any breeding program.

While card grading is unlikely to replace more traditional dog shows, many breeders use an identical thought process when evaluating their own dogs. They note strengths and weaknesses, and this helps them to balance these against one another as they thoughtfully produce the next generation. When this is done as a more formal exercise it tends to be more focused and is also more productive.

Temperament and working ability are other important key components for the success of individual dogs as well as for the utility of dog breeds (Figure 3.9). These are somewhat more difficult to assess than conformation analysis. Temperament evaluations, especially for puppies, are increasingly common across several dog breeds. The different breed groups

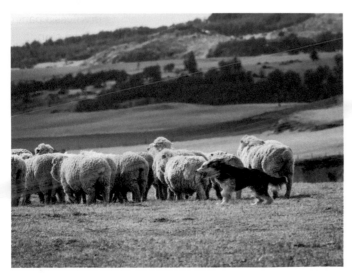

Figure 3.9 Working ability and temperament are important for many jobs dogs do. Photo by Natasha Barrios.

of dogs require very different minds to do their specific job effectively, so the broader temperament tests do need to be used wisely in some of the more specialized breed groups. Final temperament is at least somewhat conditioned and shaped by the management and interaction experience of the dog, and this must also be kept in mind when using these as an assessment tool because the environmental influences do not affect the core genome. One very constructive use of temperament tests is to help in matching puppies to specific situations to assure that puppy buyers are satisfied with their purchase.

Working ability is more complex than temperament because it is heavily influenced by management and training. Recognition of working ability can also vary and depends on the extent to which a dog is promoted and advertised. The more factors that can influence a trait, the greater the distance away from any basal genetic influence, and consequently the less closely shaped by genetic influences. It is still important to consider working ability in many breeds, because some threshold of ability is needed for success regardless of the talent of the trainer. When assessments are competitive and designate one best dog, they run into the same problem as conformation showing: selection for extremes. A top-rated bird dog might not be the best choice for a relaxing weekend hunt, and likewise a top field-trial herding dog might not fit well into the specific demands of day-to-day farming situations. A more relaxed dog can often be a better fit.

This is not to suggest that evaluating working ability is meaningless, but it is a caution that extremes can be taken beyond where they are practical. A few groups, including breed clubs or broader use-based clubs, use a certification process that is more like a baseline of ability. Above some cut-off point, a dog is certified as a worker. In many cases this approach to validation of working ability can function well to protect the working character of the breed. Rather than focusing on "the best" dog, they focus more on the rejection of "unsuitable dogs" which can then be removed from reproduction.

Performance competitions, in addition to conformation shows, can also lead to a few subtle errors in judgment. It is fairly easy in competitions to reward the biggest, smallest, or fastest dogs. This can take a population in an unhealthy direction. Comprehensive evaluation of dogs is essential to assure that sound, functional dogs continue to be bred and that they become ever more frequent in their breed. Developing evaluation schemes that assure success over long time periods is the challenge. Extremes of behavior can tip a dog over a line that is no longer useful. This can result in dogs that are a threat to others, or that are so difficult to manage that a professional trainer is required to pull the dog into a final competitive product. The key element is that the joy of ownership and partnership is then lacking.

Performance evaluation boils down to the ultimate purpose of the dog and the goal of the breeding operation. For many breeders, winning competitions is the main end-goal. In this situation, the reward for extreme performance makes at least some sense, because this is the key to winning and being the best dog. In more practical situations of daily life, an extreme dog might not be the best dog. The evaluation and rewarding of the more long-term quality of a dog in its long-term environment and role is important and is also difficult to accomplish.

The work of some breeds is so complex that no sort of independent third-party assessment is going to work well. Livestock guardian dogs are an example, where the final success in work depends on genetics, management, and specific situation. Even though external objective evaluation is impossible in these situations, breeders must be diligent and critical so that the relative ability of dogs can be known and used in making breeding decisions. Essentially, both genetics and environment have complete veto power over the final ability of the dog, so both must be considered carefully.

3.3 DNA-Based Testing

DNA tests are now available through many testing services, including both private and public sources. They are an attempt to document an animal's genotype, which then predicts what it can contribute to its own offspring. Genotypic tests only need to be performed once during the entire lifespan of the dog because the individual dog's DNA does not change over time. An advantage of genotype testing is that it is possible to test puppies prior to eight weeks of age. This helps greatly in placing puppies in the correct home when the knowledge about any mutations they carry is an important consideration.

For many genes, the results come back, locus by locus, as "clear," "carrier," or "affected." This sort of nomenclature is especially used for diseases or abnormalities caused by recessive alleles. "Clear" in this context means "non-carrier." Breeding "carrier" to "clear" will never produce "affected" puppies, only "clear" and "carrier" puppies. For many mutations, puppies can be certified as "clear by parentage" by direct marker tests if both parents have tested clear and parentage is verified by DNA testing.

Genotypic tests include those that directly detect the specific mutation, as well as those based on linked marker tests that only identify a sequence near the gene of interest. Linked marker tests are typically developed relatively quickly once a disease has surfaced and been recognized. In most situations, further research leads to the development of a direct mutation test for the same disease or locus. One general recommendation for several tests is to submit them to the laboratory where the test was originally developed. That specific laboratory is the most likely to be diligent to trouble-shoot the test for potentially misleading results.

Recent advances in DNA testing are powerful, stunning, and constantly changing. Many breeders only poorly understand the mechanisms behind DNA testing, and this can greatly limit the constructive use of the results of genetic testing in decision-making. Various assumptions lie behind these tests and their results, and some of these can lure breeders into a false sense of security by viewing the whole endeavor as more absolute and simpler than it actually is. DNA testing is powerful and useful but needs to be used wisely.

Most DNA tests are based on a specific change in a specific gene for a specific trait. Coat color and specific genetic disease traits are good examples. This approach links genetic changes to specific outcomes. It works well in most situations but involves a few assumptions that limit its application to others. One common assumption is that a single specific, documented DNA change is the only one that causes a specific trait. This is often true in one individual breed, but across multiple breeds or breed groups it is not always a valid assumption.

One example is the chocolate or liver color in dogs (Figure 3.10). The specific genetic change that results in this color varies from breed to breed, and some breeds have multiple

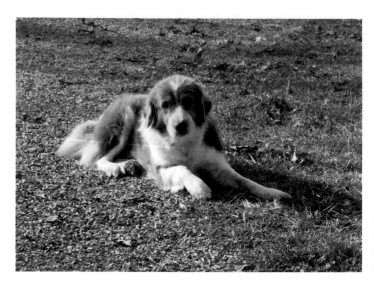

Figure 3.10 Liver colored dogs are due to one of several different recessive mutations. Photo by DPS.

numbers of these alleles. Fortunately, this is now well known, but before many of the changes were documented it was possible to encounter dogs with the chocolate color, but with a negative genetic test for the color. This is because the test can only pick up variations that have been previously documented, so new variants are therefore likely to be overlooked. The lapse in accuracy is likely to be temporary because the lag time between discovering new variants and documenting their specific mutations is becoming shorter and shorter.

The phenomenon that multiple different changes in the DNA sequence can lead to similar outcomes indicates that DNA results need to be used at least somewhat cautiously. This is especially the case for rare breeds that have different origins than most common breeds. However, glitches can even happen in more numerous breeds. The key here is that "a" cause for a disease or trait may well not be "the only" cause for that trait. As more and more mutations are identified and linked back to specific traits, the temptation is to assume that the explanation for all occurrences has been found. It is always safer to assume that genetic testing has failed to yield all information, despite the very important fact that it does indeed reveal a great deal of useful information.

It is wise to maintain at least some skepticism that DNA testing is revealing absolutely everything. The essential key is to constantly expect at least a few surprises from time to time. It is very different to use genetic tests to say, "this dog tests negative for these specific diseases on this specific panel" as opposed to saying, "this dog carries no genetic diseases." Unfortunately, many breeders extrapolate from the tests to assume that the dog is completely free of any deleterious genes, which is unlikely to ever be true.

The presence of potentially undiscovered but deleterious mutations has consequences when a dog's results come back all "clear." While this ideal result may indeed be true in some rare instances, in others it may simply be that the dog's mutations have not yet been documented. This can have an unintended outcome when such a dog sees wide use in breeding under the assumption that the dog has no deleterious traits to pass along. In a few generations any previously uncharacterized mutations can become common and can present real problems as they begin to be fully expressed. The flaw in the logic is the assumption that DNA testing can detect all weaknesses when that is not yet the case and may well never be.

Genetic tests generally work by targeting one specific DNA change in one specific gene. Historically the testing was done on a gene-by-gene basis. An alternative approach that is increasingly used relies on probing the entire chromosomal content of a dog for Single Nucleotide Polymorphisms (SNPs). SNPs are substitutions of one of the DNA code letters for another one. The specific consequences of this vary from change to change and gene to gene. The technique is powerful in revealing differences in genetic code between one dog and the next.

SNP technology yields a powerful sample of the entire genome of a dog. The probes are not random, so they can (and often do) include the specific single-gene changes that were covered by the earlier single-gene technologies. The changes related to specific and targeted sites are a great help in testing for specific diseases. In addition to these is the broader but less specific measurement of genetic variation across the entire genome. This adds a more general peek into the genome, and consequently the results of a SNP assay can be used in especially powerful ways.

One increasingly common use of SNP results is to document the presence of mutations in specified genes that lead to specific outcomes. This is the basis behind testing for coat-color mutations, and for many other morphologic or disease-related traits. The results can lead to very constructive outcomes if they are used wisely. These are especially valuable in managing recessive traits regardless of whether these lead to positive or negative traits. This is due to breeders being able to track the presence of the allele, even in heterozygotes where it is not expressed. The use of the SNP technology for this purpose does rely on the host of assumptions outlined above, with the consequence that new or rare variants are likely to be overlooked, even if only temporarily.

Another good use of SNP results comes from their ability to reveal the extent to which the genome is homozygous. SNP results reveal the relative lengths of the homozygous segments of the paired chromosomes. These homozygous segments are called "runs of homozygosity" or "ROH." The homozygous portions are related to inbreeding, and the length of these varies and reflects both the extent of inbreeding as well as a general indication of the previous generation in which the inbreeding occurred. Basically, longer homozygous stretches indicate recent inbreeding, while shorter ones indicate inbreeding further generations back (Figure 3.11). This is due to the consistent occurrence of crossover events between the chromosomes at each generational step, at a rate of slightly over one crossover per chromosome per generation. Consequently, each generational step tends to split up these homozygous regions into smaller and smaller segments. The ROH technique can capture that detail, which pedigree analysis can only estimate.

The runs of homozygosity are a direct and accurate measure of the effects of inbreeding. This contrasts with a pedigree analysis, which is based only on averages and cannot provide a glimpse into what has actually occurred. A good ROH analysis can be quite useful in managing rare breeds or rare bloodlines, because it is possible to directly minimize inbreeding even within a cohort that comes from a single litter because some littermates will be more homozygous, while others are less homozygous. This is because of the way chance works

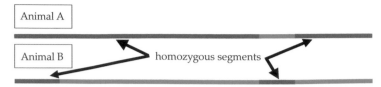

Figure 3.11 Runs of homozygosity between members of the pair of chromosomes are useful and accurate indicators of inbreeding and can also help determine the general range of generations in which it occurred. The brown segments in this figure are the homozygous segments, and the blue segments are the heterozygous segments. Animal "A" in this example has very long homozygous segments, indicating fairly recent inbreeding. Animal "B" is less homozygous, and the segments are short, indicating that any inbreeding was minor, and several generations removed. Figure by DPS.

out in populations as the chromosomes segregate and cross over at every generational step. DNA testing services increasingly offer this sort of analysis for breeders. It can be confusing to breeders when the ROH analysis results in different levels of the COI within a single litter. The COI, in this case, is based directly on measuring the ROH, and this can be expected to vary from individual to individual in any litter. The COIs across littermates are usually close to the same general value but can and do vary with some individuals being more homozygous and others less so.

It is fairly common for the ROH to arrive at a different COI than a pedigree analysis would produce. Specifically, the estimate of inbreeding from ROH is often lower than the pedigree suggests. This is especially true for dogs that are selected as superior, and therefore as candidates for reproduction. This phenomenon relates back to the basic biology of inbreeding depression. Animals that are less inbred (homozygous) are very likely to have vim and vigor, superior to their more inbred (homozygous) relatives, and are therefore more likely to be selected as candidates for further evaluation as potential breeding stock. This general bias can play out in interesting ways across an entire population. There is a tendency for the least homozygous animals, even within a cohort of full siblings, to be selectively retained as superior candidates for breeding.

3.4 Selection Decisions

Most breeders of purebred dogs strive to constantly improve their dogs for specific traits while staying within the constraints of breed type and purpose. This requires selection of breeding stock. Selection is based on evaluations. Selecting animals for reproduction is a careful balancing act that involves a whole host of very different issues that can often pull in different directions. Conformation, temperament, behavior, pedigree, breeding soundness, and genetic traits are all included. These different components work together to establish the relative value of an individual breeding dog to a breeding program.

Wise breeders know that their ideal dog is always just out of reach and that defining this ideal is influenced by current performance standards or trends within their individual breed. It is important to always be evaluating whether the current trend is something that is in the best interest of the health of their breed and whether the trend is going to have a lasting impact moving forward. Planning well in advance and evaluating the possible outcomes of how each pairing will influence multiple generations into the future allows a breeder to adjust as necessary, all the while maintaining their preferred type of dog and seeing improvements in each generation.

Breeders that sell potential breeding stock benefit when they have very specific genetic goals for their program. Future breeders who purchase these animals also benefit. Defined genetic goals are the best way to assure that the desires of both buyers and sellers can be met. In addition to the evaluation of individual animals, other things to consider are the numbers of individuals in the breed, the genetic diversity within those individuals, as well as specific health problems within the individual breed. These considerations all need to be at the base of decision trees that guide a breeding program.

Candidate dogs should be classed into categories of "ideal" and "less than ideal." Remember that some moderate dogs that don't tick all the "ideal" boxes can still be good long-term choices for a breeding program that has very targeted goals. In many situations the retention and use of moderate dogs is prudent, despite the temptation to insist that every dog be excellent or ideal. The use of moderate dogs can indeed be the important factor that makes or breaks a breeding program in ways that an elite individual dog may not be able to.

Dog breeding is complicated, and true experts in the art are rare. No dog is perfect because each is a balance of stronger and weaker points. While some weaknesses should indeed have veto power over a dog being used for breeding, it is almost always more constructive to try to achieve a balance of strengths and weaknesses in a pair of breeding dogs by matching any weakness of one dog with a strength in the other.

To achieve balance, the results of the various evaluations need to all be considered together to determine the best use of any candidate dog. These can include:

- conformation scores (such as hips)
- performance results (show or other)
- temperament tests
- genetic testing for cosmetic traits
- genetic testing for disease traits
- pedigree evaluation for rare or common bloodlines
- genetic or pedigree indications of inbreeding and kinship.

In only very few cases should any one of these have complete veto power over the rest of them. This does not mean that all caution should be thrown to the wind, because weaknesses are serious and have consequences for dog welfare. Generally, though, strengths in one dimension can be played off weaknesses in another dimension and by this strategy the weakness can be improved in the next generation (Figure 3.12). For example, the weaknesses of one parent (set of hocks, for example) might be balanced by a mate with stronger, truer hock conformation. Or a productive and useful animal with an off-type ear could be mated to a mate with a more typical ear to try to correct the type faults while maintaining all the other more positive traits that the dog might have.

Note well that only rarely is a fault corrected by mating to the opposite fault. For example, mating a dog with hocks that are too straight to a dog with hocks with too much angle is

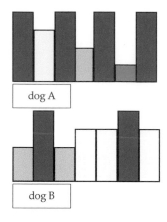

Figure 3.12 The bars in this figure represent different aspects of a dog that can be included in a selection decision. Short blue bars are weaknesses, tall brown bars are strengths, with gold and pale intermediate. In this pair, the weakness of dog A is balanced by the excellence of dog B, and none of the other traits overlap for weakness. This is an example of complementing the weaknesses of one dog with strengths in another. Figure by DPS.

very unlikely to produce a litter of puppies with hocks that are sound and true. Trying to balance faults with opposite faults is usually very disappointing. Balancing weaknesses with a mate that is ideal for the trait is a much surer path to success than attempting to balance a weakness with an opposite weakness. Balancing characteristics can be especially useful when planning the mating of two specific dogs. The weaknesses of one should be matched with strengths in the other. The goal is the production of puppies that are stronger than the weakest parent.

An important detail is that dogs arrive in litters, rather than as individuals. In most cases these littermates will all be full siblings, being produced by one sire for the entire litter. From a population genetics standpoint, the puppies are roughly equivalent to one another in their potential for contributing to the population structure of the breed. This implies that selection, even if fairly minimal overall, should at least be applied at the level of a litter to assure that the superior members of the litter reproduce, and not the inferior ones.

While only rarely should any single specific fault always veto a dog's role in breeding, it is also true that selection does need to occur. To breed sound and serviceable dogs, breeders need to be very clear-eyed about faults in their dogs, their relative severity, their influence on dog welfare and purpose, and the way that the weaknesses fit in with the weaknesses and strengths of other dogs. No dog is perfect, but nearly all dogs have at least some positive attributes. Balancing these is the goal of successful breeding.

Dogs that are selected for reproduction usually strike a balance between various factors (Figure 3.13). Only a very few dogs will be exceptional across all of these. Those few have exceptional conformation, perfect temperament, great behavior, no hidden genetic flaws, and good fertility. Such dogs, if they come from rare bloodlines, also have the added benefit of bringing genetic variation to their breed. Most dogs are going to play these issues off one another, with compromises between strength in some of them and relative weakness in others. The balance of these, and how they fit together, is important when making decisions to use a dog for reproduction, and just exactly the role that the individual dog should have in reproduction and contribution to the breed.

Balancing the various factors that lead to dog selection takes dedication and creative thought, because they interact with one another in various ways. For example, a dog from a very common bloodline should only be used if the physical structure is excellent (this

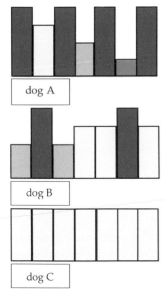

Figure 3.13 Dogs used in breeding programs are a balance between many factors, generally with both weaknesses and strengths. The weakness in dog A is counterbalanced by multiple strengths, but this dog should still be used only cautiously in a breeding program. Dog B, in contrast, balances moderate weaknesses with significant strengths and can be used more safely and more broadly. Dog C might well be overlooked in many breeding programs, but the consistent (if moderate) strengths and the lack of weaknesses make this dog a safe mate for a wide variety of other dogs. Figure by DPS.

includes hips and elbows along with everything else), the temperament is stable and good, and the genetic health traits are good or exceptional. In contrast, a dog from a rare line that has some good attributes may well be allowed to be lacking in some of these other criteria, although always with the caution that rarity, in its own right, does not excuse major flaws. While it is easy to simply leave it at "major flaws should not be routinely used for breeding," the unfortunate truth is that "major flaws" often means very different things to different breeders. What might be acceptable to one breeder might be of grave concern to another. These differences in philosophy can generate heated disagreements among breeders.

One characteristic that should likely be ignored in most situations is "convenience" or "affordability." The easy availability of any specific dog does not necessarily make it a good choice for reproduction or as a good match for the proposed mate. All the other factors in mate selection are much more important than convenience in making breeding decisions.

Not every mating has the same goal or tactic, even though the obvious and intended outcome is a litter of puppies. Understanding that the puppies in the next generation might have different destinies helps breeders to shape their kennels by planning which dogs will contribute in which specific way. Each dog has a different importance in respect to its genetics, productivity, conformation, and contribution to the genetic structure of the population.

In a very real sense, each dog has its own role and potential. Realizing this is central to making genetic progress at the population level. Likewise, each dog and each mating have a different importance to the overall breed. For example, the single remaining female of a unique foundation strain needs to be used much more strategically than a female of a more common or composite bloodline even if they are otherwise similar for conformation and production levels. Likewise, a sole remaining male of a rare strain might be allowed minor faults to a greater degree than a male of a common strain to assure that the positive attributes of the rare strain are not irretrievably lost.

Each mating should be evaluated as to its likelihood for producing puppies that are strong and healthy, as well as how the puppies produced will fit into the population as potential breeding animals. The main mindset to use when evaluating breeding animals is to figure out just how their offspring, both male and female, will fit into the population and be used, whether that is for breeding, show, performance, or sport. One reason for mating might be to balance bloodline representation.

While not all puppies may see wide use in reproduction, each nonetheless carries with it expectations for at least some constructive use. Especially for rare breeds, specific matings should always consider the quality of the animals as well as their ancestral background. In some situations, one or the other of these factors can be the most compelling, and there is no set rule to establishing which of these is more important in any specific situation.

Good breeders spend years identifying breeding stock that is worthy of reproduction. Dog evaluations are strategic ongoing tasks that are never finished! The overall merit of any potential breeding dog is based on the breed standard, the dog's intended use, and on the dog's temperament. These components are all essential. Not only is the individual dog's genetic makeup important, that of its predecessors can also play a crucial role. This is especially true when long-term management of genes is the goal.

Prudent breeders consider the management of a dog that is a breeding prospect to be starting from day one and extending on throughout its life. These factors are directly related to the genetic side of selection and management and are essential to the success of any breeding program. Other factors relate to veterinary care, general health management, and life management. These factors are equally important, and ensuring their high quality is essential for final success.

3.5 Selection Consequences of Reproductive Protocols

One aspect of assessment that is generally not considered is a direct assessment of the animal's reproductive capacity. This can include parameters of normal reproduction such as age of puberty, but also includes any assisted reproductive technologies. Any intervention into a natural cycle of mating, pregnancy, and whelping can have unintended consequences if not carefully evaluated. Nearly every aspect of reproduction is under genetic control. In most situations the control is polygenic and not due to single alleles. A few consequences of some of the reproductive interventions are important to consider (Figure 3.14).

Age of maturation and development can vary from animal to animal, bloodline to bloodline. This rarely causes problems, but in certain circumstances needs to be a trait considered in selection. The age of puberty is one important factor. If ignored, it can become increasingly delayed in a bloodline. For males, the delay can also be in the descent of testes which can lead to cryptorchidism if allowed to progress too far in a bloodline. For females, the result can be delayed or erratic estrus.

Testicular size is related to levels of sperm production in males. It is also related, within a bloodline, to ovarian size. While this may seem trivial, larger gonads produce larger volumes of gametes, which means larger litter sizes. If gonadal size is allowed to diminish from generation to generation the eventual outcome can be rare, small litters.

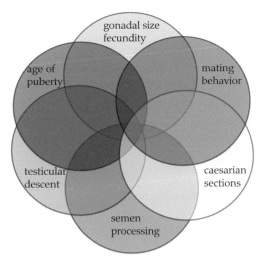

Figure 3.14 Successful reproduction depends on several underlying factors. Each of them is under some level of genetic control, which must be considered in selection decisions. The small area where they all overlap is where reproduction is the most problem-free. Figure by DPS.

The entire process of mating and conception also has several control points along the route. Artificial insemination can completely bypass these if its use is not carefully considered. The biggest risk of problems comes when artificial insemination is used to circumvent a problem with natural conception rather than for some other reason related to convenience or availability. Artificial insemination can eventually result in diminished expression of mating behavior or other adverse behaviors. It can also lead to diminished selection for normal reproductive tract anatomy and function.

The process of freezing semen can also have unintended genetic consequences because not all males will be equally successful. In the early days of freezing semen for dairy bulls, many of the candidate bulls failed to pass the threshold for the freezing process. Over time the percentage of failures diminished because genetic selection had removed those bulls from the reproducing population. The genetic contribution to the breed was then limited to only those bulls whose semen could be successfully frozen. This is a subtle but important issue and can be repeated in other species if caution is not used.

Caesarian section versus natural whelping can also have important consequences. In the American situation, some breeds favor large forequarters, small hindquarters, and short broad heads. Breeders of some of those breeds have resorted to timed caesarian section instead of natural whelping. This completely removes any need for the breed to be able to whelp naturally and can eventually lead to a situation where natural whelping becomes impossible and caesarian section then becomes an essential component to the future of the breed.

While these can all be consequences of assisted reproduction, the conclusion is most definitely not that all assistance is detrimental. Each of the techniques that can be used to assist are appropriate in some situations. Each must be used wisely, especially when broadly used across an entire breeding population. Otherwise, they run a risk of unforeseen genetic consequences for animal well-being and function.

3.6 Key Points

- Dogs can be evaluated through different means, each of which yields different information.
- The most accurate selection is possible when there is a close match of evaluation and genetic basis for a trait.
- Genetic tests are useful, but do not provide the whole story.
- Genetic tests for specific alleles can overlook new or rare mutations.
- Genetic tests for runs of homozygosity can help manage inbreeding.
- Genetic tests can be misused.
- Conformational evaluation is useful, but environmental influences complicate its accuracy.
- Final dog selection depends on:
  - o pedigree evaluation
  - o genetic testing
  - o conformational evaluation
  - o ability in desired task.
- The consequences of any assistance for reproduction need to be carefully considered.

CHAPTER 4

Managing Genetic Traits

Dog breeds face several different genetic challenges. These can be broadly broken down into two main divisions.

- Specific individual genetically controlled conditions (this is the topic of this chapter).
- The structure and organization of the breed as a genetic pool, as reflected by the inter-relationships and numbers of dogs and bloodlines (this is the topic of the next chapter).

Individual genes and population structure differ from breed to breed. Each must be given careful consideration in any breeding program that aims to serve the long-term future of the breed as a valuable addition to human and canine life. Simply adding numbers of dogs to a breed may be only marginally helpful. For example, the addition of dogs that all come from a single bloodline can bring a few risks. Such a strategy not only increases the distribution of the strengths of the line, but also increases the distributions of any of its weaknesses. Most breeds need careful management of their population structure, including the management of specific genes that cause disease or weakness.

4.1 Selection and Genetic Drift

The management of genetic traits is based on the ways in which the frequency of alleles can change from generation to generation. Change of frequency occurs in a few ways. Some of these are more deliberate than others, but it is important to understand all of them to manage the genetics of breeds and individual dogs. (Figure 4.1).

The most deliberate way to change genetics is through selection. Selection changes the genome of the breed by retaining or diminishing specific genetic variants. Selection is the most secure way to accomplish genetic change over time and is the one way most under the control of the breeder. Selection is used to decide which dogs reproduce, and it is wisest to do this very thoughtfully.

A second way in which gene frequencies can be changed is through genetic drift, which is a consequence of the random passage of alleles from generation to generation.

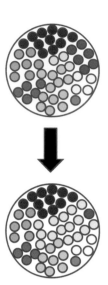

Figure 4.1 Gene frequencies can change from generation to generation. In this example, the light blue has increased, the brown has decreased, and mid blue has almost disappeared altogether. This can be accomplished either deliberately by selection, or by the chance that dictates genetic drift. Figure by DPS.

However, genetic drift can result in the loss of rare alleles. For example, if an allele occurs in only 1% of the dogs in a breed, the passage of that allele to the next generation is very likely to fail entirely by chance and not because of selection. This becomes important in small populations that have rare alleles. Small population size constrains rare alleles to being present in very few dogs, and therefore they risk being lost completely because they fail to be passed along from generation to generation. Single alleles that are likely to suffer this fate are usually the ones that control qualitative traits such as color or coat type, although this is also true for alleles that contribute to traits such as ability and temperament. All these traits can be lost to drift unless they are carefully monitored and considered by breeders.

4.2 Philosophies for Managing Genetic Traits

Genetic traits are the primary building blocks that combine with the environment to produce the final dog. One way to think of this is that the genetic component sets out the basic range of possibilities, and the environment then works on these to shape the final product. Genes set the potential, and then the environment determines whether that final potential is reached. Because they are the basic building blocks, genetic traits should be managed carefully to assure that sound and useful dogs are the final product of a breeding program.

Genetic traits include many that are positive and highly sought in a breeding program. Genetic traits can also be negative and can be shunned by breeders. The character and consequences of what are usually considered to be negative traits vary considerably. Diseases or conformational weaknesses that are caused by genetics are clear examples of negative traits. Other traits fall into a more middle ground, such as undesired colors, markings, or other cosmetic flaws that do not really impair the soundness or function of the dog.

Unfortunately, there is no clear dividing line between the negative traits that are more serious and the ones that are somewhat trivial. Individual breeders will draw that line in different positions, and often defend their stance vehemently.

Philosophies behind the breeding of dogs can vary, and some of them bring with them especially deleterious consequences. One extreme is "anything goes, and every dog deserves to reproduce." Some observers refuse to acknowledge this philosophy as "breeding" because it does not provide for improvement or even maintenance from generation to generation. It is an extreme followed by very few, and perhaps they should be called "multipliers" instead of "breeders." This extreme philosophy leads to a complete lack of selection, with no room for progress in the control of weaknesses or genetic disease. The breeders at this end are hopelessly optimistic. They think that nearly every dog (especially the ones they own!) is perfect.

At the other extreme are breeders that are hypercritical. They refuse to breed a dog that has any weakness or that carries any gene for genetic disease. This extreme view puts undue pressure on the population structure, because very few dogs (if any) can pass this hurdle.

Somewhere in between these two extremes is a balanced point where progress is possible, while also ensuring that a sufficient number of dogs participate to ensure sufficient levels of genetic variation to maintain the breed's population (Figure 4.2). Genes have importance not only for the individual dogs, but also for the breed in which they occur. Considering both levels is essential for their successful management, especially if the goal is to have sound and functional purebred dogs going forward into the future.

An important issue for individual breeders as well as breed clubs is to decide when, or if, certain traits or certain alleles should ever have complete veto over the reproduction of the dogs that have them. On a superficial level it is easy to say that no breeder should allow the reproduction of a dog with any gene that contributes to disease or weakness. At the practical level this quickly reduces the pool of eligible dogs to a negligibly small number that can barely sustain any breed in a meaningful and long-term way. The consequence of this is that broad and absolute rules almost never serve to wisely shape breeding programs.

Somewhere between "anything goes" and "strict rules" lies a point that serves breeders well and serves dogs and dog breeds well. Exactly where that balance point resides varies from breeder to breeder. Breeders generally do best when they carefully evaluate their own individual philosophy towards animal breeding and revisit it from time to time to accommodate any changes that may need to be made as situations change and as more information becomes known. A consistent philosophy allows breeders to make consistent

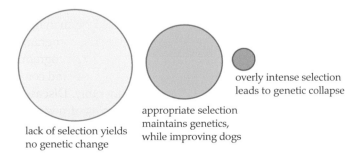

lack of selection yields
no genetic change

appropriate selection
maintains genetics,
while improving dogs

overly intense selection
leads to genetic collapse

Figure 4.2 Too little selection can lead to absence of any genetic change, while too much can lead to eventual collapse of genetic variation needed for variability. Figure by DPS.

decisions that serve their breeding program well and helps them in their attempt to meet their individual goals.

Regardless of an individual breeder's final choice of guiding philosophy, it is wisest to learn various ways that alleles can be managed constructively in a population. Full knowledge allows breeders to choose among the many options that are possible. Wise management includes many options besides drastic removal of all negative alleles. The specifics are strongly influenced by the mode of inheritance of the trait. The genetics behind most traits fall into a few general categories. It is useful to know the general category of the genetic mechanism for a trait because this affects how breeders can and should manage them.

Many traits are caused by single genes (Figure 4.3). These are the easiest to manage. How these genes occur in and travel through populations is the key to their successful and constructive management, which is heavily influenced by their specific mode of inheritance. Other traits fall into the category of polygenic traits because they are caused by several genes working together, with a range of expressions related to the specifics of the allelic variants that are present. These polygenic traits are much more complicated, both in terms of expression and in terms of techniques to manage them in a population. A subgroup of these are the polygenic threshold traits that are caused by multiple interacting genes, but that are only present if some threshold of alleles is present and below which there is no expression. These can be the most challenging to manage.

4.3 Managing Single Gene Traits

A wide variety of traits are controlled by single genes. These include traits of weakness or disease, as well as more cosmetic traits. Most single-gene traits are shared across several breeds, although some do have a limited occurrence in only one or a handful of breeds.

Color comes to mind as one obvious trait that can be important in many breeds or breeding programs despite its relatively minor role in the well-being of dogs. Color is controlled

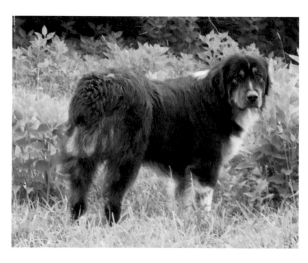

Figure 4.3 Single-gene traits, like the short tail of this Karakachan dog, are the easiest to manage. Photo by DPS.

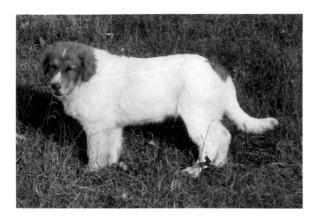

Figure 4.4 Karakachan dogs with red marks are becoming more common in this breed that is often black and white. Photo by DPS.

by relatively few genes, and as a result is relatively easy to control (Figure 4.4). It is important to remember that "relatively easy" does not necessarily mean "100% of the time." Color preferences in several breeds are a good illustration of the ease of managing single genes, and the powerful consequences of selection. Some colors that were once rare in some breeds have become very common through intense selection over very few generations. The wide array of colors currently available in Dachshunds, for example, has resulted from taking alleles that were once rare in the breed and making them more frequent through the power of selection. A similar pattern is occurring in French Bulldogs, a breed in which rare or unusual color combinations are especially popular currently. Karakachan dogs with red and gold markings have also become more frequent due to selection by breeders.

The advantage of working with single genes is that they are relatively easy to track, identify, and manage. This is increasingly true in today's world, even for recessive alleles, because the technology to accurately identify many allelic variations has become routine through the easy availability of DNA tests. The ease with which single alleles can be documented has important practical consequences. Single alleles can be easily tracked through sequential generations, and breeding practices can be tailored to assure their expression if that is the desired outcome, or to assure that they are not expressed if that is instead what is desired. Even though recessive alleles avoid expression in heterozygotes they can still be tracked in this way. The specific pairs of dogs that are mated can be manipulated to either keep recessive alleles hidden or to facilitate their expression by producing homozygous dogs.

The specific mechanism of the tests for various alleles is an important detail, and these vary from test to test. Most of the available tests directly detect the specific genetic change that is responsible for the allele of concern. This sort of direct test is very accurate for a specific allele, although it can lull the user into thinking that "an answer" is "the only answer." That assumption is sometimes made in error. The key detail is that loci can have multiple alleles, each due to a different genetic change even though all of them can lead to a similar final phenotype. A failure to detect one of the alleles through genetic testing does not mean that the others are absent. This subtle fact can sometimes cause problems when DNA results become a major way to select breeding dogs while other factors are ignored.

A few tests do not detect the specific change in the DNA that causes a specific allele, but instead detect a change that is located close to the allele. These tests can be a bit problematic.

They only function accurately if the linked two sites are close together on the chromosome, and if the change at one site is always associated with the change at the other. Over many generations the possibility of a crossover event between the two linked sites assumes 100% correlation to be decreasingly likely. While these tests work accurately for many traits of interest, they must be interpreted carefully. When a crossover does occur the test loses its ability to accurately identify the allele that is of interest to breeders. After a crossover event the test becomes inaccurate not only for the dog with the crossover, but also for all its descendants.

4.3.1 Recessive Alleles

Recessive alleles, by their very definition, are only expressed when an animal has two copies of the same allele. Expression requires two copies, and those with only one copy are silent carriers with no expression. The mathematics of the behavior of alleles in populations is such that the frequency of the silent carriers is much, much greater than the frequency of the animals that express the allele in the homozygous state. For example, if a recessive allele is expressed (homozygous) in 4% of a population, then the frequency of silent carriers is a whopping 32%. While selection may target the homozygotes (either favoring or shunning them) it needs to be sensitive to the real consequences of actions that affect the numerous heterozygotes.

One way to manage recessive alleles is to eliminate all copies of the allele. This can be done by testing the DNA of all breeding dogs and then removing all those carrying the allele (Figure 4.5). This simplistic approach has at least two consequences. One consequence

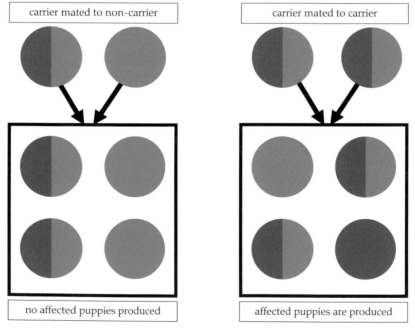

Figure 4.5 Mating a carrier of a recessive allele to a non-carrier (left mating) will not produce any offspring that express the recessive allele in the phenotype. In contrast, mating two carriers (right mating) will produce normal animals, carriers, and puppies affected by the allele. Figure by DPS.

is fairly obvious: if the allele is not present (because breeders have eliminated it), then it can no longer produce the affected phenotype. This sounds harmless if the goal is to indeed eliminate the phenotype. However, the alleles responsible for the phenotype are often present in some families and absent in others. Removing all of the carriers shifts the whole population away from the families that have the allele and towards the ones that lack it. Selectively removing all of the carriers thereby not only shrinks the gene pool, but also shifts its structure. For breeds with small population sizes this can severely damage a structure that may already be perched on the verge of extinction.

An alternative strategy is to focus on the phenotype rather than on the allele itself. Under this strategy, dogs could be tested, and then the stipulation could be put in place that carriers of the allele would not be mated to one another. This strategy works to eliminate expression of the phenotype, while not eliminating the allele that causes it. This can be seen as a subtle or trivial difference, but it has radical consequences for the population. This strategy allows carriers of the allele to pass along their good qualities while at the same time ensuring that they do not actually produce the undesired phenotype. Including the carriers in the breeding population can be important to the future of the breed, even if the one specific phenotype is not desired. Over time it is also possible for breeders to selectively retain the non-carrier offspring of carriers, which gradually eliminates the allele while not simultaneously removing all the other genetic contributions that carriers might be able to make. In most situations the breed benefits if that process of removal is accomplished relatively slowly.

Single genes related to disease traits obviously have important consequences for animal welfare. They can be managed creatively and successfully in small populations by using the same strategy outlined above. Nearly all breeds have at least a few recessive alleles related to genetic disease, and the underlying principles work equally well for all of them. In the case of disease-causing recessive alleles, the animals with two copies of the allele either fail to survive at all or face a very compromised life. In this situation "doing nothing" is not a satisfactory option for their management. Further complications arise when the recessive allele causes a disease that is only manifested in older dogs that may have already reproduced. In that situation homozygotes can escape early detection by anything other than a genetic test. Relying on phenotype alone is an inadequate strategy for managing such traits, and in any event cannot completely reveal all carriers of a recessive allele.

Even though disease-causing recessive alleles should be a target of negative selection, it remains true that removing all of the carriers of the allele can have drastic negative consequences for population structure. Following that strategy can result in entire families of dogs being removed completely from the breed, or at least decreased in numbers. Many breeds cannot withstand that loss and maintain genetic viability for other traits. Basically, targeting the single allele can end up ruining the rest of the genome of the population that is so necessary for animal soundness and well-being.

The dogs with only one copy of a recessive disease-causing allele are perfectly normal and can lead normal lives (Figure 4.6). Consequently, there is little concern for any welfare or well-being issues. With these alleles it is often wisest to encourage testing of dogs, but then to impose the single restriction that carriers are not mated to one another. This strategy instantly assures that no affected dogs will be born, despite the presence of the allele

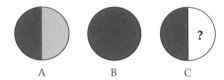

Figure 4.6 This is an example of three individuals, all three of them express the normal dominant brown trait. Tan is recessive, and none of them express this trait. Genetic testing can separate out carrier A from noncarrier B. Individual C is not tested, and therefore it cannot be determined if this animal carries the recessive or not. C can only be safely mated to B, and not to A. Figure by DPS.

in the breed. A modification of this strategy will be more practical in some breeds: test all males, and then require that carrier males only be mated to females that have been tested and are noncarriers. Noncarrier males can be safely mated to any female, including females that have not undergone the genetic test, because noncarrier males have no risk of ever producing affected puppies.

Results of genetic tests do influence the demand for, and relative economic value of, breeding animals. This is an important issue for single-gene disease traits and is especially true in today's world of easy access to genetic testing for a wide range of alleles. Animals that are carriers, even though they are phenotypically normal, are usually less economically desirable than animals that are free of the alleles. Some level of this preference is going to be nearly impossible to avoid, and if taken to the extreme this will have the same consequences for the population as a strictly imposed rule-based approach to eliminate carriers. In some situations, it is wise to ensure the use of certain carriers. This approach might require certain incentives if market pressures resist the use of all carriers.

In many cases it is best for overall population management to assure that animals of rare bloodlines are used for breeding even if they carry deleterious alleles, provided those alleles are carefully documented and carefully managed. Using such animals assures that the breed does not lose the remaining balance of the carrier dogs' genes that offer so much to breed viability. The key point is that carriers can be safely used, with the single stipulation that they are not mated to other carriers. In succeeding generations, the non-carrier offspring can be selectively retained. This is slower than the immediate removal of carriers of an allele but is an effective strategy that allows carriers to contribute to the genetic future of the breed without passing along the disease coded for by their deleterious allele. It is vitally important to realize that carrier animals have many more genes than the single one that is the target of this test. Breeders need to balance the potential negatives (which can usually be fairly easily managed) against the positive contributions that the rest of their genome can make. Removing animals from reproduction removes not only that single allele, but also the rest of their genetic makeup.

A contrasting situation faces breeders that are interested in ensuring the production of homozygotes for recessive alleles that are desirable. Many of these relate to color, but other examples do surface from time to time. DNA testing can help in this situation because it can help to locate heterozygous carriers that do not express the phenotype, but that can produce it. This strategy often increases the number of potential breeding dogs, especially when contrasted with strategies that can only identify carriers by a pedigree of having a parent with the expressed trait.

A problem that underlies the goal of producing homozygotes of rare recessive alleles is that this often requires some level of inbreeding. This needs to be managed carefully to avoid potential problems. Tracking heterozygous carriers using DNA analysis is a particularly good way to do this. This allows breeders to find heterozygous carriers of the allele that are unrelated to current breeding stock. Matings can then be arranged to the unrelated noncarrier, which minimizes inbreeding, while also ensuring the production of homozygotes in a portion of the resulting litter. Testing can also be used for evaluating puppies from a carrier and an unrelated noncarrier. The carrier puppies from such a litter can then be identified and selectively retained so that they can in turn be used in the breeding program. This not only assures that they carry the desired recessive allele, but also helps breeders to be able to minimize the level of inbreeding that will assure its expression in homozygotes.

4.3.2 Other Single Alleles

Recessive alleles are not the only disease-causing alleles. Alleles with other modes of inheritance are a bit more complicated to manage. Some alleles produce phenotypes that are desired when that allele is present in one copy, but that are deleterious when two copies are present. An example of this is the allele for "bully" whippets that have a dramatic increase in muscle. In heterozygotes the allele causes a slight increase in muscle and speed, which gives them an advantage in racing. When two copies are present the result is very thick muscles, with an odd look as well as less speed. In this situation the heterozygotes do have an advantage, but it is generally best to avoid mating them together to avoid producing homozygotes with the undesired phenotype.

The mating of two bully whippet carriers together produces offspring that are (on average) 25% normal, 50% slightly affected, and 25% bully. Mating a bully whippet carrier to a normal whippet produces offspring that are 50% normal and 50% slightly affected. The result is that both types of mating give only 50% of that desired heterozygous phenotype, but the "bully carrier" to "normal" mating produces no bully puppies. The only way to assure 100% production of the slightly (and positively) affected whippets is to mate a bully whippet to a normal one. While this does produce 100% of the desired heterozygous phenotype, two dogs have produced it, both of which lack that phenotype. This can have subtle consequences because it is not possible to have fine-tuned selection within the desired phenotype when neither parent exhibits it.

Similar issues arise with the production of merle dogs. The desired merle phenotype is heterozygous (Figure 4.7). The homozygotes that lack the allele have full expression of black or liver color and, in most breeds, these are either black, black and tan, liver, or liver and tan. The homozygotes that have two copies of the merle allele are very pale, and most often have hearing or visual problems, or both. This is a welfare issue and is used to argue against the use of homozygous merle dogs in a breeding program, even though they would be assured of 100% production of merle puppies when mated to a non-merle dog.

There are only a few examples of diseases caused by dominant alleles. These are the easiest to manage because they can be eliminated based on phenotype alone. This does depend on the age of onset of signs. Even with a dominant allele, wisdom can dictate that

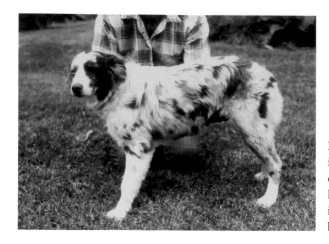

Figure 4.7 Merle dog color is an interplay of dilute and dark patches of fur, a phenotype caused by a heterozygous condition for an incompletely dominant allele. Photo by DPS.

the occasional animal with the allele should be mated despite the risk of affected offspring. Such a mating may rarely be necessary to avoid losing important genetic traits other than the one that is deleterious. Such cases are rare but are very important when they arise.

Dominant alleles that cause late-onset disease are especially challenging because expression may be delayed past the usual time of selection for reproduction. Relying on phenotypic classification alone is problematic with this class of diseases. Genetic testing can be very helpful in charting out a strategy because it can identify affected animals before they actually express the disease.

One advantage for breeders wanting to manage single-gene traits comes from the fact that modern technology allows the alleles to be tracked and managed effectively. The time interval from first discovery of a disease-causing allele to the development of a final diagnostic test has become shorter and shorter as DNA technologies have become more readily available and more powerful. The result is that breeders now have many tools at their disposal. Figuring out just exactly how to use the results of these technologies for the betterment of the breed is a challenge and is much more complicated than a simplistic approach of simply and quickly eliminating all copies of any deleterious allele.

As with most technology, testing for single alleles is "value neutral." The outcome depends entirely on how the results are used. It is important to note that once an allele has been removed from a breed, it is gone for good and cannot be recovered. This includes genes that might be out of favor today, but tomorrow could find a renewed and favorable demand. While this is unlikely to be the case with disease-causing alleles, it remains true for some of the more cosmetic traits. In most situations, effective breed management should at least attempt to save the entire breed package, regardless of current trends in demand (Figure 4.8).

Genetic testing for single-gene disease traits has become strongly adopted by dog breeders of many breeds. Most dog breeds have at least a few diseases related to single genes, and breeders logically have a desire to eliminate the production of disease-prone puppies. In many breeds this has led to a breeder culture where animals for reproduction are all tested, and all carriers are eliminated. This can have very negative long-term consequences through the drastic reduction in the reproducing population of the breed.

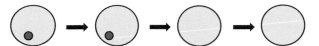

Figure 4.8 This single allele (the brown dot) is passed along through the first generation to the second, but then fails to make it to the third generation. That makes it unavailable for the fourth and all succeeding generations. Figure by DPS.

A second consequence is more subtle. As animals are eliminated for carrying identifiable alleles, it has also happened that the survivors carry other alleles that are in fact deleterious but for which there is currently no test, or no previous knowledge of the syndrome they cause. The newly encountered disease then becomes a widespread problem, all because of over-eager use of testing and removal for the other deleterious alleles encountered previously.

Nearly all individual animals have at least a few deleterious alleles. One estimate is that they each have at least four or five. This means that effective management relies on much more than a "test and eliminate" mentality, and more on developing ways to manage the genes for successful outcomes that avoid expression of deleterious alleles. The key point is that selection programs based on single genes can have fairly quick results. Those results can be positive and encouraging, but unless the selection programs are wisely implemented, they also have potentially devastating long-term consequences. These can be detrimental to a breed and its future viability. It has also often been the case that the initial "absolute truth" of a genetic situation in animals has later proven to be much hazier than initially thought, with the consequence that early attempts at wise genetic management have been proven to be just the opposite. Genetic uniformity can have devastating effects, as evidenced by the Irish Potato Famine where the uniformity of the potato varieties led to collapse of this important crop as one disease eliminated production of the one variety that had been so extensively planted. Complete genetic uniformity comes with real risks!

4.4 Polygenic Traits

Several traits are controlled by many alleles at multiple loci. These are called "polygenic traits." The environment of the dog plays an especially significant role in the expression of many of these traits. Most performance traits fall into this category, with characteristics such as speed and size serving as good examples. While the single-gene traits are largely a question of "yes or no," the polygenic traits are more a question of "how much?" These two situations are very different and require different strategies for their effective management.

The fine details of many polygenic traits are being increasingly uncovered, including some of the specific underlying genetic changes responsible for such traits. Among these details are the fact that some alleles contribute more to the outcome than others. This complicated situation is very different from that involved in the single-gene traits, where it is possible to accurately determine a dog's propensity to pass along a specific allele. Polygenic traits evade that level of accurate detail, partly from the genetic mechanisms involved but also because of the environmental contributions.

One of the most historically perplexing polygenic traits in dogs is hip dysplasia. It can serve to illustrate a number of important points about polygenic traits more generally. Hip dysplasia can be understood at a number of levels. The disease is progressive over time, and it can be measured in different ways and at different times. Each of these has consequences for diagnosis and management of hip dysplasia.

One approach is to focus on the endpoint of dysplasia, which is an unsound, or even crippled, dog. This is the underlying reason for selecting against hip dysplasia and is an important endeavor for the welfare and utility of dogs. The unsoundness is related to arthritic changes in the hip, which are in turn a consequence of increased laxity of the hip joint. The overall cascade of events is something along the order of:

- genotype which leads to …
- lax hip joint, which leads to …
- arthritic changes, which leads to …
- joint pain and lameness.

In addition to the general framework of physical changes is the job the dog does (athlete versus sedate house dog) and the underlying resistance of the dog to experience pain or discomfort. Some dogs with minimal changes are profoundly lame, some dogs with relatively severe changes show little outward sign of the disease (Figure 4.9).

Exactly how to move forward to reduce the incidence of hip dysplasia is therefore complicated. At one extreme is a view that limits any concern about the disease to the expression of obvious lameness. This view would tolerate dogs with physical changes but with no outward sign of lameness. The opposite extreme would be to focus on the physical propensity of the dog to develop changes that can lead to lameness, even should this only occur in a few dogs. This second view eliminates dogs that would never experience any of

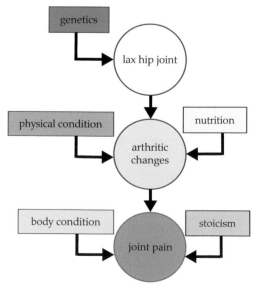

Figure 4.9 Hip dysplasia is the result of a cascade of changes that result from the environment affecting the basic genetic starting point. Figure by DPS.

the consequences (lameness) of dysplasia. It does, however, also do a better job of eliminating the production of those that might possibly become lame. These two are philosophically quite different, and either one could be held by some breeders as a perfectly logical approach.

Beyond discussion of the genetic, environmental, and inherent behavioral aspects of dysplasia lies the basic progression of the disease as it develops from hip laxity to arthritis to unsoundness. Each of these three can be a logical point of measurement and evaluation. An important detail is that the key to strong and effective genetically based control programs is that the measurement and evaluation should be as closely related to genetic potential as possible. Hip joint laxity is fairly strongly correlated with genetic influences, which makes this factor a preferred site for evaluation.

The next step down from hip laxity is arthritic change. It is one more step removed from the underlying genotype, and consequently the environment intervenes and complicates assessment. A dog with lax hips but maintained in a fit, trim body condition is likely to have minor arthritic changes when compared to a dog with the same degree of laxity that is kept roly-poly fat and in weak physical condition. Through the influence of environment, it is therefore possible to mask (or accentuate) the genetic potential.

The final stage of hip dysplasia is lameness or unsoundness. At this level, yet more factors emerge. The environment remains a strong influence. To this is added the individual dog's response to pain or discomfort as well as its relative level of activity. Some dogs are simply more stoic than others and exhibit little pain in the face of a level of arthritic changes that might cripple a less stoic dog.

The important detail is that each step removed from the initial factor (genetic potential) introduces more chance for the environment to mask the effects of the genes. Each step down the cascade reduces the power of the evaluation for genetic potential. The most accurate place to measure the genetic potential is therefore the earliest point, which in the case of hip dysplasia is the joint laxity itself because it is unrealistic to directly measure the various alleles that contribute to the outcome. Then, of course, the next question is to decide what to do about it.

At the outset it is important to understand that selecting against hip dysplasia has had variable results. In some situations, this is due to fairly casual attention to this trait on the part of breeders. This, predictably, leads to little progress. In other situations, the attention has been quite high, and the selection has been strict, but the results have still been disappointing. This reflects the complexity of the trait with genetic and environmental interactions, as well as when and how to measure the trait. In addition, the two main evaluation methods, OFA and PennHip, do not yield identical results. OFA evaluations are based on changes in the joints, while PennHip is based on the degree of laxity in the hip joints. At least some studies indicate that some dogs rated by OFA standards as normal do have degrees of hip laxity that are likely to lead to osteoarthritis as the dog ages (Figure 4.10).

With hips, and other conformational traits, a tension exists between deciding if a dog is "better than the rest" or simply "good enough." Hip evaluation results can be used in various ways. One way to use results is a "within breed" evaluation that places the dog's scores against the scores of others in the same breed. This can have a subtle effect of imposing the assumption that tighter hips are always better in every situation and for every breed.

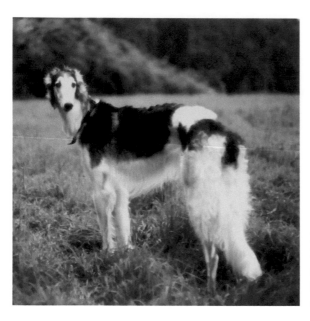

Figure 4.10 Breeds vary in their risk for hip dysplasia, and recommendations need to be tailored to specific breeds. Sighthounds, such as the Borzoi, are at especially low risk. Photo by DPS.

Hip laxity is better understood as a sort of threshold trait, so that below some value of laxity, "tighter" basically does not offer any greater protection against the dog developing hip dysplasia.

Especially in tight-hipped breeds (sighthounds are an example), most dogs are "good enough" to provide minimal risk of the negative effects of hip dysplasia. In that situation, discarding dogs because they are looser than the breed average can remove dogs that could well make a positive contribution to the breed, while at the same time not actually reducing the already minimal risk of dysplasia. While this is true, it is equally the case that hip laxity, even in a tight-hipped breed, cannot be completely ignored because that approach risks an eventual loss of soundness if the hips become increasingly lax as the generations proceed.

In contrast, the laxity scores in a relatively loose-hipped breed can be used effectively to assure that hips become tighter as the generations proceed. This will reduce the incidence of hip dysplasia over time. The threshold for this selection criterion in many breeds is generally a distraction index of 0.30 or lower, because this indicates hips that are tight enough to avoid any degenerative changes nearly always. This, as with most recommendations, should not always be used as an absolute rule. In general, scores around 0.40 are usually at mild risk of dysplasia. Many breeds have dogs in the range of 0.30 to 0.40 that have positive traits for the breed, while also posing minimal threat of unsoundness. Any firm cut-off point is therefore unwise without considering other factors of importance to the breed. A lack of strict rules might seem too permissive, but this is far from advocating an "anything goes" policy where dysplasia is ignored and where no progress is possible.

Using any type of hip scores needs to be put into context of the whole dog. Even with the availability of a good and objective test, a relatively lax score should not necessarily be an automatic veto over reproduction in all situations. Dogs with loose hips might well have other traits that could serve their breed well, although such dogs must be used wisely, cautiously, and sparingly. This is not a blanket recommendation to throw all caution to the wind, because lax hips, or any other faults, are a serious impediment to dog welfare and well-being. That said, an automatic "cull" decision based on any one test can take dogs out of the breeding population despite their many positive traits. While this is true, it is equally true that many owners of breeding dogs are overly optimistic of a dog's positive points and are too dismissive of the dog's weaknesses. The result is a risk of using inferior dogs for breeding.

In this example, dogs with lax or loose hips should never be mated together. However, at least some of them have served their breeds well by being mated very selectively, and minimally, to dogs with tight hips. The goal is to constantly improve weaknesses rather than spreading weaknesses around. The mistake to avoid is the mating of two dogs with similar weaknesses, and to avoid the mating of a dog with multiple serious weaknesses. While no specific and absolute cut-off of laxity is wise for any breed, it remains true that tighter hips are less likely to develop dysplastic changes than are looser hips. Breeders should pay attention to this fact.

A few other techniques are available to manage hip dysplasia for large populations that have good control over breeding and evaluation. Guide dogs and service dogs are often bred in controlled programs. In this situation it is possible to rate nearly all dogs that are produced in the program. Those results provide sufficient information to produce an "estimated breeding value" (EBV) that indicates an individual dog's propensity to produce puppies with either lax hips or tight hips. The EBV figures are derived from collateral relatives of the individual dog, and this enhances the accuracy of understanding the individual dog's genetic potential. Across dogs with identical PennHip scores, some will be less likely and others more likely to produce puppies with greater laxity. This degree of information is rare in most breeding populations, because it requires fairly large numbers of fully evaluated dogs in order to be accurate. The strength of this technique is that it gets closer to genetic potential than the other techniques do. Fortunately, valid and successful breeding decisions can be based on the laxity figure itself. The EBV just takes that to the next level of accuracy so that progress is even more rapid, with the usual warning that rapid progress can remove too much genetic variation if done unwisely.

A key concept in this regard is that polygenic traits are basically "how much" rather than "either/or." This means that although breeders can expect surprises along the way, they can also rest assured that dogs with fewer of the offending genes are less likely to produce the unwanted defect than are dogs with more of them (Figure 4.11).

4.5 Polygenic Threshold Traits

Several traits take the complexity of polygenic traits to a next level that is even more complicated. These are the "polygenic threshold traits." This refers to the fact that several genes are indeed involved, but that the trait itself is not expressed until some bottom threshold of numbers of alleles is achieved. These traits are difficult, because dogs that are just below the threshold for expression will not express the trait but will still be at a fairly high risk of being able to pass it along to their offspring. It is impossible, from phenotype alone, to accurately identify those dogs that have very few or none of the alleles and to separate them from those that have several but are just below the threshold. Obviously, these two classes

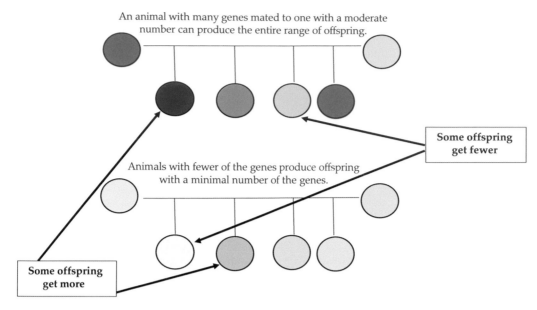

An animal with many genes mated to one with a moderate
number can produce the entire range of offspring.

Some offspring
get fewer

Animals with fewer of the genes produce offspring
with a minimal number of the genes.

Some offspring
get more

Figure 4.11 Polygenic traits can be imagined as shaded circles, with darker circles representing animals that have relatively more of the alleles that influence the trait and paler circles representing animals with fewer of those alleles. Each animal can contribute different amounts of shading (alleles), but never any more than it has to offer. Taking the contribution of any animal to zero is unrealistic in most situations. The more alleles that are present (the darker color) the more that they are likely to be passed along to offspring. Some offspring get more of the alleles, some get fewer. The process is one that is dictated by chance and probabilities. Figure by DPS.

of dogs have very different consequences for a breeding population. As the technology for developing genetic probes advances it may one day be possible to achieve a higher level of detection for the alleles that lead to these problems.

The more usual polygenic traits (those without a threshold) can be managed fairly well by wise pairing, even of dogs that are affected to some degree. In the case of polygenic threshold traits, the inability to accurately identify dogs just below the threshold means that a somewhat different selection practice may be needed (Figure 4.12). Below the threshold the breeder is basically "driving blind" because it is not possible to know the fine details that would help make fully informed decisions.

For these traits, it is wisest to remove any affected dogs from breeding. Among the polygenic threshold traits are several structural cardiac defects. It is fairly easy for nearly everyone to agree that these should be removed from reproduction because cardiac function may be compromised. In addition, dogs that are first-degree relatives of an affected dog are also likely to have several of the offending genes even if they do not reach the threshold necessary for expression of the defect. In this situation it is wisest to also remove these first-degree relatives from breeding, even if they themselves lack the defect. This is drastic, and a recommendation that can be modified in some specific situations. The key point is that first degree relatives of affected individuals are very likely to have a number of alleles that are just below the threshold, and therefore risk transmitting them to the next generation.

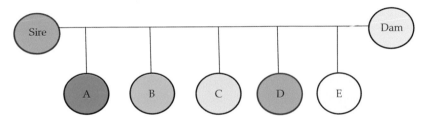

Figure 4.12 Polygenic threshold traits are challenging because dogs below the threshold do not express the trait. In this example, paler blue indicates dogs with fewer of the genes responsible for the trait. The sire, puppy A, puppy B, and puppy D all express the trait. The dam, puppy C, and puppy E do not express the trait, but both the dam and puppy C have sufficient alleles to contribute to its expression in the next generation, while puppy E has minimal chance of doing so. Figure by DPS.

This recommendation will seem too severe to many breeders. As with all rules, hypothetical cases can be built for at least some exceptions to the rule. However, when dealing with polygenic threshold traits breeders do need to be aware that these alleles can lurk unexpressed in fairly large numbers, and they therefore warrant fairly strict selection to be sure they do not increase from generation to generation in a breed or bloodline. When they do increase, the number of affected animals will drastically rise, and control measures will then be very difficult.

4.6 General Gene Management

Managing genes is important, and unfortunately the fine details can vary for each allele. The main issues to consider include:

- mode of inheritance
- frequency of the allele
- time of onset of the phenotype caused by the allele
- desirability (or not) of the allele
- availability of an accurate genetic test.

Regardless of the mode of inheritance, the breeder's task is to try to locate the alleles of interest in the population, and then to manage them effectively so that they are either increased (if desired) or decreased (if not desired). This can involve some creative thought that combines the mode of inheritance, the trait in question, and the long-term breeding goals. The identity of the alleles as discrete bits of information that can be tracked from generation to generation helps this process along greatly because it allows breeders to either facilitate or eliminate the expression of the allele without necessarily eliminating the allele itself. This realization allows for inclusion of a wider range of breeding candidates than a strategy based more narrowly on directly eliminating alleles.

The cultural environment in which dog breeding occurs has a considerable influence on what breeders do and how they do it. In some cultures, the breeding of dogs has become highly regulated, whether directly by governments or by breed clubs or associations. In other situations, the breeding of dogs is basically not regulated at all. Restrictions on dog selection vary widely, and the discussion above is largely under the assumption of minimal regulation. This is not to imply that this is necessarily the best situation. It is, however, the situation where breeders have the most opportunity to make independent decisions and therefore have the greatest degree of individual responsibility to see that sound dogs are produced and that breeds are kept genetically viable.

The long-term goals are sound dogs and sound breeds. While those two goals may seem identical, they are not. In some cases, they pull in opposite directions, and wise decisions can be difficult as it is necessary to make a compromise between the two for the long-term benefit of both dogs and dog breeds.

4.7 Key Points

- Effective management of alleles depends on the mode of inheritance of a trait.
- Effective genetic management may not always lead to complete removal of an allele, even those with detrimental effects.
- Knowing which dogs have which alleles can help in managing the alleles to either avoid expression, or to assure expression.
- Age of onset of expression of genes is an important factor in timing evaluation and selection of evaluation tools.
- Traits with high levels of environmental modification are especially challenging.

CHAPTER 5

Maintaining a Breed or a Bloodline

Maintaining a bloodline, or an entire breed, requires close attention to population structure. This is especially true for any population where genetic isolation is required. Genetic isolation can be absolute, as is the case with dog breeds, or somewhat leakier as is often the case with individual kennels that maintain a bloodline within a larger breed. Genetic isolation needs to be a bit leakier where population numbers are low, even if some degree of genetic isolation is desired.

The three goals for long-term breed or bloodline management are:

- purebred breeding within the breed's gene pool
- production of sound dogs, including their structure, genetics, temperament, and function
- maintenance of a genetically sound breed.

Successful strategies for breed or bloodline management always balance the support of these goals to ensure they can be continued long into the future.

Breed maintenance depends on the individual matings that occur between members of the breed. The challenge is to keep in mind what happens two to three generations on into the future when planning a single mating. Long-term management of the genetics of populations is essential to this process and is basically the management of levels of inbreeding. Wise genetic management of populations assures that benefits of inbreeding can accrue from its positive aspects while avoiding the risks that can arise from its negative aspects. Inbreeding (and the declines in vigor and health that it often brings) is most likely to occur when it becomes inevitable as the only option within a breed or kennel. This happens when all dogs are related to one another.

Long-term management of inbreeding ideally assures that outcrosses are available for every animal within the population, whether this be a single kennel or an entire breed. Inbreeding levels can be managed to ensure they stay within safe limits by occasionally outcrossing to unrelated animals, with the stipulation that these outcrosses be from within the same breed. Managing breeding programs to assure that unrelated outcrosses are possible over the long term is challenging and requires close attention to a host of details.

An important detail is that mating to an unrelated animal immediately takes the offspring's level of inbreeding back to zero. This is true even if one parent has a coefficient of inbreeding that is quite high. Coefficients of inbreeding only reflect the degree of relationship between the parents, so if they are unrelated, the resulting coefficient is zero.

5.1 Genetic Bottlenecks

Genetic bottlenecks occur when only a few individuals of a breed remain (Figure 5.1). The original, larger population becomes narrowed to only a few animals. Bottlenecks are a drastic form of over-representation of specific animals. These few individuals then become the founders for the entire future of the breed. Bottlenecks reflect the fact that each animal can only have up to two alleles at a single locus. This translates into the principle that fewer animals inherently have fewer options for maintaining genetic diversity, even under the unrealistic assumption that they are heterozygous at all loci. This general trend becomes even more severe when all those animals are related to one another.

Bottlenecks reduce genetic variation and can constrain the viability of a breed. A short bottleneck happens when a single constricted generation of small numbers is followed by rapid expansion. This is much less harmful than a long bottleneck that lasts for several generations. Long bottlenecks are especially damaging as alleles are more likely to be lost to genetic drift, resulting in a drastic reduction of genetic variation over several generations.

Bottlenecks are important in the fate of breeds. While "avoiding bottlenecks" sounds easy, in practice it can be quite difficult. To avoid bottlenecks it is necessary to have adequate numbers of unrelated dogs. Those dogs, logically, are going to vary in quality and potential, and the tendency is to discard all but the most elite of the dogs. While it is wise, and usually necessary, to have a good and strict program of selection based on quality, it is also true that exceptions can be imagined for nearly every rule that would automatically remove specific animals from any reproduction.

Bottlenecks in dog breeds often occur due to intense and severe selection in favor of only the most elite males, as determined by only a limited array of assessments (Figure 5.2). Elite males sire the subsequent generation, and selection once again pulls out only a few elite sons. As this proceeds from generation to generation, the process slowly eliminates genetic

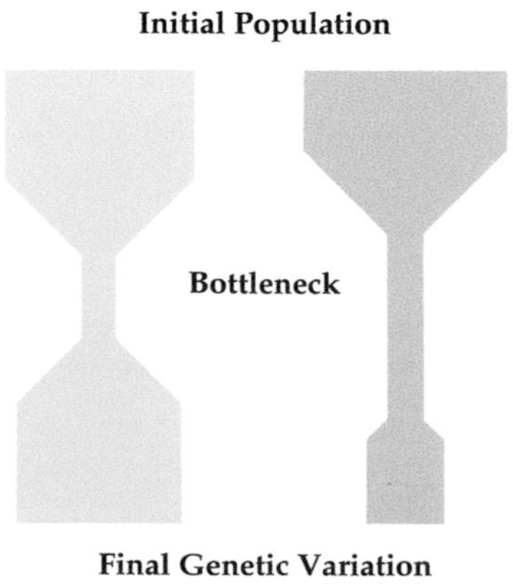

Initial Population

Bottleneck

Final Genetic Variation

Figure 5.1 Bottlenecks occur when population numbers decrease. When they decline for only a few generations (as shown in the blue diagram) the effects are much less severe than when they persist for several generations (as shown in the tan diagram). The longer or narrower the bottleneck, the less genetic variation survives. Figure by DPS.

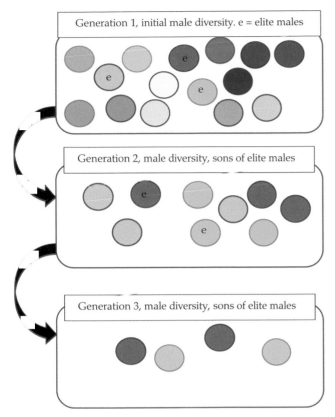

Figure 5.2 Use of only a small portion of elite males sequentially robs a population of diversity as the generations proceed. Figure by DPS.

variation. The breeding strategy that strictly limits reproduction to only the most elite dogs, assures a generation-by-generation decrease in genetic variation.

Selection of dogs for breeding can affect bottlenecks. Selection, in most situations, is based on a variety of assessments that balance one against the others. It is important to remember that certain individual dogs can provide genetic variation in ways that are just as important for the long-term survival of a breed as are any elite dogs identified by their performance, conformation, or other quality. The role or place of an individual dog in the genetic structure of the breed therefore needs to be added to the list of potential assessments that can influence the decision to include dogs in the reproducing population.

The misuse of assisted reproductive technologies such as artificial insemination can also easily lead to bottlenecks. These technologies are most commonly used to provide wider access to an outstanding individual than would be possible through natural reproduction. The consequence is an over-representation of that outstanding individual because he essentially swamps the breed with his own genetic material at the expense of everything else that is available.

Alternatively, and importantly, assisted reproductive technologies can be used wisely for targeted goals that can be very helpful in providing genetically sound and viable structures for rare breeds. For example, semen can be saved from a wide variety of dogs as a wise strategy that assures that their genomes are present for future use. This can be especially useful when selection targets change over time and breeders want to return to characteristics that were more common in the past.

5.2 *Monitoring Effective Population Size*

Effective population size is a relative measure of the number of truly different genetic individuals in a population. This refers specifically to individual dogs that are used for reproduction, so it excludes the many dogs that never reproduce. Effective population size is influenced by several factors. For example, a group of ten full siblings represents a lower number of genetic individuals than a group of ten unrelated dogs does because the genetic variation is much lower in the family group than in the non-family group.

Effective population size can be a useful estimate of future inbreeding trends because low effective population size indicates a future in which all animals will be related and therefore all matings will be inbred. Effective population size is related to specific expectations in the increase in inbreeding coefficient per generation.

Effective population size is most simply expressed as:

$$1 \div \text{effective population size} = \{[1 \div (4 \times \text{number of males})] + [1 \div (4 \times \text{number of females})]\}$$

The numbers of males and females in the formula are the numbers of reproducing males and females. The mathematics of this can be overwhelming, but the core of the idea is that the sex with the lowest population tends to determine the effective overall population size. For most breeds this means males. The most obvious consequence of this, if effective population size is to be boosted, is that effective breed management usually involves using more males than would be absolutely necessary if the only consideration were the number of females a male can manage to successfully mate with. Genetic consequences dictate a different answer for the number of males that should be used when compared to the number required by animal management considerations.

Effective population size is dramatically affected by the sex ratio. A breeding population of 50 animals could be 40 females and 10 males, which gives an effective population size of 32. If the population were 25 males and 25 females, then the effective population size is 50. Constraining the population to have relatively more males raises the effective population size dramatically. The influence of different sex ratios is illustrated in Table 5.1. If the total

Table 5.1 Effective population size relative to proportions of males and females in a population of fixed size. Reducing the number of males dramatically reduces the effective population size.

Number of males	Number of females	Effective population size
25	25	50
10	40	32
5	45	18
1	49	4

population size is kept constant, then the more equal the sex ratio, the greater the effective population size.

Two additional important points about effective population size are presented in Table 5.2. The first is the outcome of using different numbers of males on a constant number of females. As the number of males decreases, the effective population size decreases rapidly. The second is the effect of increasing the numbers of females mated to only one male. Raising the number of females even two- and three-fold in that situation does very little to increase effective population size. The lesson here is that sex ratios for effective breed management need to be carefully considered, and they usually involve using more males than might seem logical for strictly reproductive purposes.

The equation given previously for effective population size is oversimplified and a longer, but more accurate, equation also includes the time interval from parent to offspring for each sex, as well as the degree of relationship between animals. These are important issues for effective population size but are difficult to account for in most situations. The broad brush of the simplified equation serves to drive home the most important points that are also most subject to influence from breeder decisions.

The important summary is that the effective population size is generally lower than the census would suggest. Any shared ancestry among breeding partners (especially in recent generations) takes that number still lower. The effective breeding population size is almost always much smaller than the outright census. Unfortunately for breeders of rare breeds, it is impossible to easily capture all the information for an accurate determination of effective population size. The level of detail needed to arrive at an accurate answer is overwhelming. The simplified equation is useful in highlighting the importance of sex ratio, especially in rare breeds, but it is important to note that the number generated by this result is likely to be a relatively optimistic one. The true effective population size is generally even lower than the figure predicted by the simplified equation.

Effective population size is a more critical factor for breed survival in rare breeds than it is for breeds with large populations, because inbreeding in rare breeds is more likely to be widespread throughout the entire population. The principles of effective population size are a compelling reason to keep track of different bloodlines within rare breeds so that breeders can assure that outcrosses are available to each animal in the breed. No specific guidelines can be offered to suggest a ratio between census and effective population size,

Table 5.2 Consequences of sex ratio and population census on effective population size. When small numbers of males are used, even dramatic increases in numbers of females have minimal effect in increasing effective population size.

Number of males	Number of females	Total population	Effective population size	Increase in inbreeding coefficient per generation
30	30	60	60	0.82%
9	30	39	27.6	1.8%
3	30	33	10.9	4.6%
1	30	31	3.87	12.9%
1	60	61	3.934	12.7%
1	90	91	3.96	12.6%

as this is a complicated biological concept and oversimplifying it leads to a false sense of security about the true genetic composition of purebred populations. Breeders should monitor their breeds closely to assure that outcrosses are available within the breed. Breeders should be diligent to keep different bloodlines viable and secure as insurance against future needs.

5.3 Inbreeding and Loss of Diversity

Inbreeding has several important consequences. One is inbreeding depression, which refers to the decline in vigor of inbred animals as compared to outbred animals. Inbreeding usually diminishes the overall vigor of the resulting animals, as well as their reproductive success. Inbreeding depression in dogs often shows up as decreased fertility rates and decreased litter sizes. This occurs at variable rates in different populations so that the practical significance of this phenomenon varies. Exceptions to the general rule do occur, but they are just that: exceptions. Focusing on those successful examples overlooks the overwhelming long-term risk that uncontrolled inbreeding often brings to a population.

A second and important consequence of inbreeding in small populations occurs when it combines with genetic drift and selection to reduce genetic variation (Figure 5.3). The result can strengthen and accentuate predictability. As animals become more genetically uniform, they also tend to become more similar in looks and performance. Predictability is the hallmark of pure breeds, and so this can be a good consequence of the reduction of genetic variability. The downside is that overall levels of genetic variability are essential not only for population health, but also in providing the raw material for selection and improvement. Highly inbred populations may lack sufficient variability for selection efforts to make any progress in performance levels.

Even though some lines of some breeds withstand inbreeding very well, inbreeding depression is a widespread and well-documented phenomenon. All breeders should manage their populations to ensure that problems of inbreeding can be avoided in the long term. Breeds should be managed so that every animal within the breed has an outcross available. This strategy assures that a "back door" escape is available to the breed should inbreeding depression become evident. Inbreeding and its consequences can then be quickly remedied by resorting to an outcross. The situation to be avoided most is the

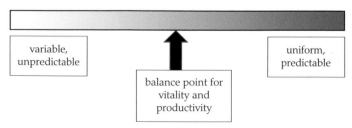

Figure 5.3 Genetic variability tugs in an opposite direction to uniformity. Uniformity assures predictability, which is one of the goals of purebred breeding, but due to decreased vitality the actual point along which uniformity becomes a problem can be important. Figure by DPS.

one in which all animals within a breed or bloodline are so closely related that inbreeding becomes inevitable.

Genetic variability and genetic uniformity play tug of war. Populations at one extreme are so variable that they are completely unpredictable as to type and production. Populations at the other extreme are so uniform that vigor diminishes, and genetic selection is impossible because all animals within the population are so similar to one another. Most breeds lie between these extremes and must be managed so that the benefits of predictability are not lost to diminished vigor on the one hand, and so that enhanced vigor is not gained at the expense of low predictability on the other hand.

5.4 *Monitoring Inbreeding*

Monitoring the generational increase in inbreeding is especially important for small, isolated populations such as dog breeds. Exactly how the inbreeding is distributed across a breed can vary, even in populations that are made up only of inbred animals. Two examples help to illustrate the importance of the distribution of inbreeding:

- All the animals are inbred, but not to the same individuals within the breed. In this situation it is possible to lower the inbreeding coefficient in subsequent generations by selectively mating to unrelated animals.
- All the animals are inbred to the same individuals. In this situation no unrelated matings are possible and corrective measures are not available to decrease inbreeding coefficients.

The consequence of these two different distributions of inbreeding within a breed is that the specific character of the inbreeding is of as much concern as the overall degree of inbreeding. If the inbreeding is occurring in different directions (to different individuals) then the breed is less precariously perched than if the inbreeding is all occurring to the same few individuals across the entire breed.

The degree of inbreeding across the entire breed is important, and equally important is the degree in individual animals. To track this detail most effectively, it is necessary to evaluate the degree of inbreeding with respect to several different founders instead of using a single average across the entire breed. This can be done by evaluating kinship among the animals of the breed. Kinship is the relative closeness of relationship between two animals and is the hypothetical inbreeding coefficient of offspring that the two would produce if mated to one another (Figure 5.4).

The overall degree of kinship of one individual animal to all other individuals in a breed can be important. The ideal is a detailed individual-by-individual analysis to assess the range of kinship from one individual to all their potential mates. An example is to consider two hypothetical situations where the overall degree of kinship to a specific individual (usually male) is 25%. In one situation the range of kinship across individuals might be 20% to 30%, which indicates that all potential mates are related to the individual in question. In this situation all potential matings are inbreeding. In the second situation the kinship could have a range of 0% to 30%. In this second situation, outcrosses are still available because unrelated animals are in the population. In the first case, they are not available, and the

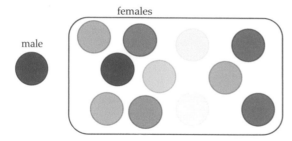

Figure 5.4 Kinship measures the degree of relationship between an individual dog and its potential mates. In this figure, darker potential mates have higher kinship, paler ones have less kinship. This can help drive breeding decisions, although each of these mates is logical in some situations and for some specific breeding goals. Figure by DPS.

breed has hit a true bottleneck regarding that individual animal because all matings must now be inbred to that individual.

The key concept is that kinship is just as important as a coefficient of inbreeding. As long as some kinships are zero, outbreeding is possible within the population. Kinship is a bit tougher to track than the coefficient of inbreeding, and it can also be slightly more challenging to visualize. Despite the difficulty in understanding and using it, it is a useful tool in breed management.

5.5 Inbreeding Within Individual Kennels

Degrees of inbreeding levels are likely to be higher within an individual kennel than they are across an entire breed. This is largely due to the use of relatively few males in most kennels, with retention of breeding stock from a single or only a few sires or outstanding dams. Over several generations of closed kennel breeding this strategy can lead to fairly significant inbreeding within a single kennel. This can be one of the sources of the uniformity that is usually desired in the dogs produced but must be done with forethought.

In most breeds, inbreeding within a single kennel is of little threat to the overall genetic health of the breed. This is true because other kennels are either being outbred or are being inbred to different individuals. As long as the inbreeding is not the result of the same few individuals across the entire breed, then the breed is relatively safe and does not risk losing much genetic variation. The reason for this is that one inbred line can be linecrossed to a second unrelated inbred line, and all the inbreeding that is built up vanishes in the next (linecrossed) generation. A backcross to either parental line will assure that inbreeding is once again occurring, so wisdom and close management are needed if the goal is continued assurance that outcrosses are available to every animal in the breed.

5.6 Inbreeding Within Breeds

Inbreeding is much more problematic when it is uniformly distributed across an entire breed rather than within separate kennels. When inbreeding is uniform at the breed level it is nearly impossible to avoid its negative consequences. If all breeders pursue the same successful bloodlines and individual animals, then the result is that the entire breed is being inbred in the same direction. This can be visualized as a circle with the tension at the boundary all being directed into the same middle point, which is usually a popular individual animal or bloodline (Figure 5.5). Over several generations the circle, which represents the

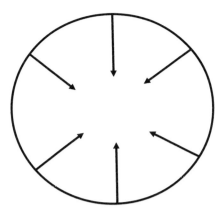

Figure 5.5 Inbreeding in a single direction across an entire breed yields a constricting gene pool for the entire breed. Figure by DPS.

overall genetic variation in the breed, becomes smaller and smaller. Popular sires or blood-lines that expand at the expense of others in the breed are common culprits for significant inbreeding problems across entire breeds. It is especially dangerous to use uncontrolled artificial insemination, as the entire breed can be mated to a handful of related sires. Such a strategy accelerates the inbreeding that occurs.

The ever-contracting inbred circle can be contrasted to the situation in which different bloodlines within the breed are being bred in different directions and to different individual animals (Figure 5.6). In that situation the inward forces are subdivided into sub-circles within the larger breed circle. The result is that the overall breed circle tends to maintain its original size without much loss and genetic variation, along with breed health.

Strategies for managing inbreeding vary from breed to breed, depending on association rules or governmental regulations. At one extreme there is no control at all over inbreeding, nor strategies for managing it. Inbreeding is unavoidable in situations where a lack of restrictions results in breeding that is concentrated on only a very few individuals. Some breeds are now reaping the unfortunate consequences of this as dogs are produced with diminished vigor. The philosophy and practice of purebred dog breeding, as envisioned over the last two centuries, have not yet fashioned a good strategy for dealing with inbreeding in

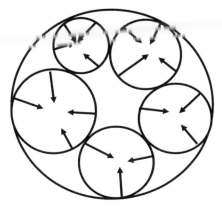

Figure 5.6 Inbreeding in various directions by concentrating it in different kennels can keep more genetic diversity in a breed than inbreeding all in one single direction. Figure by DPS.

closed populations. Over the next few decades, breeders and associations need to address this issue if the genetic heritage of breeds is not to be lost through their attrition to extinction from lack of vigor.

Many dog breeds provide very good lessons for the management of long-term purebred breeding. Dogs have a short generation interval and produce relatively large litters, so their role in this grand experiment of purebred breeding is ahead of most other species. As the standardization and closure of breeding populations was initiated over a century ago, it began a process of genetic isolation and therefore consistent, if gradual, diminution of genetic variation from generation to generation. How to manage this ever-contracting genetic variation, while preserving the very real advantages of purebred dogs, is a challenge that will require creative thinking on the part of both breeders and breed associations.

Some breed clubs may well choose to control inbreeding by limiting the number of offspring registered per animal, per year, or per lifetime. Very few breed associations use this sort of control. This tactic can be especially important when artificial insemination is widely used. Putting a limit on the number of litters an animal can produce in a year or a lifetime assures that no single animal's offspring can swamp the entire breed. One useful benchmark is that in most breeds it is unwise for any sire to produce more than 5% of the offspring in a given year. This can be a very difficult step for a breed association to take because it pits the long-term survival of the breed against the short-term economic benefit for individual breeders who have popular animals. It is, however, a very realistic goal for nearly all dog breeds, and most have already met it.

In many breeds it may not be necessary to have a formal set of rules to manage inbreeding. In most breeds it is possible to educate breeders about the bloodlines within the breed and the need to keep these going into the future. A quick analysis can usually reveal which lines are becoming rarer and which are in danger of swamping the breed. Alerting the breeders to the status of the bloodlines can boost activity within the rarer bloodlines, especially if this is matched with long-term educational endeavors on the part of the breed association about the importance of bloodlines within a breed.

Noting the production record of sires that produce offspring can help breeders to analyze the bloodlines of sire families. One way to do this is to count offspring and grand offspring for all sires. This can be done either as a year-to-year analysis, or as a lifetime analysis. The results of the analysis keep track of breeding activity for each animal, and when done by someone familiar with the breed can also track the breeding success of entire families.

For rare breeds it is helpful to have a more detailed analysis that tracks the breeding status of different family lines, especially targeting those that have few animals or are lacking animals of one sex or the other. These underrepresented families can then be targeted to be sure that they reproduce, and that offspring are recruited into the breeding population of the breed. When accomplished over several bloodlines, this approach can help to assure that each animal within the breed has an unrelated potential mate.

5.7 *Strategic Use of Coefficients of Inbreeding*

In many breeds it has become fashionable for breeders to pay close attention to the coefficient of inbreeding. Fortunately, there are many computer programs available that do this handily from pedigree information. It is an important measure but needs to be put into a broader context than simply stating that high coefficients are always bad. The coefficient of inbreeding can also be calculated from the runs of homozygosity revealed by a detailed DNA analysis. This technique provides the most accurate reflection of the actual genetic status of the dog because it is a direct measurement of a dog's level of homozygosity rather than a statistical expectation such as the coefficient of inbreeding that is derived from pedigree information.

As with most of life, the devil is in the details, and simple solutions tend to overlook real complexity that lies below the surface. One increasingly common recommendation is to simply avoid mating animals that produce a relatively high coefficient of inbreeding in the offspring. This is generally based on pedigree analysis, with all the underlying assumptions and weaknesses that this brings. The cutoff level for rejecting inbred matings varies but is often 10% or so. This sounds harmless, and even potentially good. This strategy basically avoids higher inbreeding coefficients.

A potential problem with this strategy that avoids high coefficient of inbreeding is that it can lead to breeders constantly seeking out matings that minimize the resulting coefficient. This sounds wise at first glance but can easily lead to a few unanticipated consequences. A constant drive to minimize coefficient of inbreeding has the outcome that minimally related dogs are constantly mated to one another. Over several generations this tactic essentially uses up those unrelated matings (Figure 5.7). This happens because unrelated dogs are preferentially brought together, so the resulting puppies are related to both. The eventual result of following this strategy over sequential generations is that all animals eventually

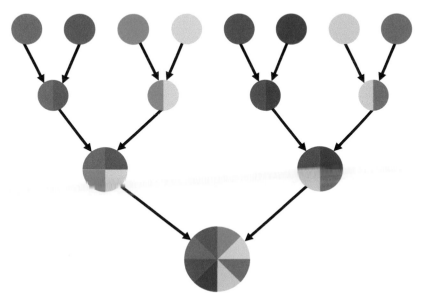

Figure 5.7 The different colors in this diagram represent different founder dogs, unrelated to one another. These are preferentially mated to minimize the coefficient of inbreeding, with the result that in the fourth generation the animals are related back to all the founders, which then assures that every mating is an inbred mating. Figure by DPS.

become related to one another. At that point completely unrelated mating strategies are no longer available. This is a subtle outcome that is not obvious to most breeders. This process of sequentially increasing kinship by using outbred matings occurs much more quickly in a breed with a small population than in a breed with a larger population.

Coefficients of inbreeding, and measurements of kinship, must be used wisely and with forethought as to how various strategies are going to play out several generations into the future. A very high coefficient of inbreeding in an individual animal is not necessarily bad as long as animals with no kinship are available. Mating animals with no kinship takes the coefficient of inbreeding of the next generation back down to zero because coefficients of inbreeding only refer to the relationship among parents. The fact that even a high coefficient of inbreeding can be taken back to zero opens many more options for future use of those animals, although this does depend on the availability of unrelated mates. In that regard, paying close attention to kinship might be more useful, if more difficult, than focusing on the much easier coefficient of inbreeding.

5.8 Combining Linebreeding and Linecrossing

One mechanism for population maintenance that can work well for a number of breeds uses the advantages of both linebreeding as well as linecrossing (Figure 5.8). Mating can be constrained so that following a generation or two of linebred matings, the animals are then linecrossed. By alternating the two mating strategies generation to generation it is possible to reap the benefits of each without experiencing too many of the negative aspects of either. This can be done by paying close attention to the management of two bloodlines but is much more powerful when more than two are involved. Such a plan does require great

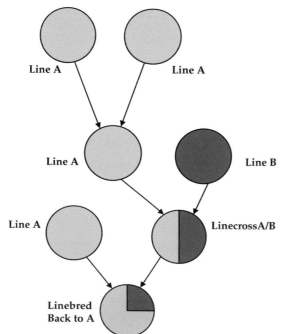

Figure 5.8 Alternating linebreeding and outbreeding in sequential generations is one way to maintain genetic variation while retaining the advantages of both strategies. Figure by DPS.

attention to detail because matings must always consider the fate of the animals several generations into the future. This can be managed so that the inbreeding stages do not result in extremely large coefficients of inbreeding, while at the same time ensuring that at least some potential mates in the population are minimally related.

Both inbreeding and outbreeding have a place in breed and kennel maintenance. Making sense of all the details of inbreeding and linebreeding can be perplexing, especially when breeding decisions must be made by breeders. Associations can help their breeders by educating them concerning the lines within the breed and the importance of these for breed-wide genetic health. Especially difficult is the very real consequence that short-term economic interests pressure breeders to all pursue the same breeding direction by trying to produce animals that fit current demand. In contrast, long-term breed viability requires that breeders maintain sufficient diversity for breed viability. Managing the tension of these two demands on breeders is a very important role for associations and breeder communities.

5.9 Inbreeding and Linebreeding to Expand Rare Genetics

Linebreeding has a few specific powerful benefits for many rare breed or bloodline conservation programs. A major strength of inbreeding, and linebreeding is the fixation of traits in a given line of animals. This can be used to good advantage in several situations. Linebreeding is a power tool that must be used cautiously and safely to assure its benefits and avoid its potential risks. Targeted close linebreeding or inbreeding is an effective strategy that can correct the under-representation of the genetic influence of rare bloodlines or specific founders of rare breeds. It can also enhance imported bloodlines that may have only come through a single sex of animal. This is often through a male imported via semen, but occasionally by a female of a rare bloodline.

This strategy involves fairly intense, if temporary, inbreeding. The rare animal can be mated, and the offspring saved. That rare animal can then be mated back to one of its offspring. The resulting puppies are 75% the influence of the original animal, but with a high coefficient of inbreeding. One advantage of dogs is that they are produced in litters, and in this inbred litter it is possible to select out the best and most vigorous puppy to be used in the next step, which is to use the animals of this generation as outcrosses to other lines. The initial step of very close inbreeding cannot be continued for multiple generations in a row, but it does succeed in making a single rare animal's genetics much more broadly available.

The key to success with this strategy is to use it only as a rescue strategy for a rare bloodline, or to limit it to truly outstanding individuals. This strategy depends on the past efforts that dedicated breeders of purebred dogs have made to assure the availability of truly excellent animals. Every breed benefits from having such breeders and such animals. It is the long-term dedication of individual breeders that provides these distinctive genetic packages that are so useful for others to build upon. Each breed, and each generation within the breed, needs breeders dedicated to safeguarding the genetic heritage and productive potential of the breed. In contrast, if this strategy is used on weak or average individuals, the risks of inbreeding depression outweigh the potential benefits of salvaging the genetic material.

5.10 *Managing Contributions of Individual Animals*

It has already been stressed that every animal should have a potential linecross within the breed to assure the breed's genetic health. This requires attention and careful planning; otherwise, all animals of a breed can become related to one another. This usually occurs through the over-use of individual excellent animals. Especially in dog breeds, certain individual animals have become over-represented, to the extent that it is nearly impossible in some breeds to find linecrosses (Figure 5.9). When certain animals become over-represented, other animals become under-represented, and the breed risks losing their genetic contribution. When individuals become over-represented, it means that the breed has lost variability, and could be in danger of losing the genetic variation essential for long-term survival.

In situations where multiple sires are used in a single year, or for a single generation, it is important to recruit replacements from each sire rather than from one of the sires (Figure 5.10). This ensures that genetic diversity is retained. It can be tempting to deviate from this strategy when the sons of one of the sires are better than the others. However, constraining the choice of replacement males to include the sons of all sires, rather than only a single one, allows selection of the best son to be combined with genetic breadth that can lead to long-term success of the breed.

Another way that individuals become over-represented is the "popular sire" phenomenon. The popularity of a given male may be such that many breeders use only him, or his sons. This can easily swamp a breed and is a major problem in some purebred dog populations. Show ring success is commonly the underlying reason for a sire's popularity. In many cases breeders have discovered only in later generations that a genetic problem has been identified with some such popular sire. By that time eliminating the problem has become

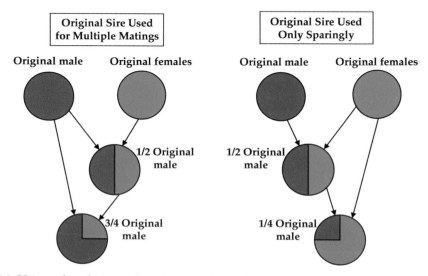

Figure 5.9 Using a foundation male only sparingly results in a very different pattern of genetic distribution than using him in multiple generations. Figure by DPS.

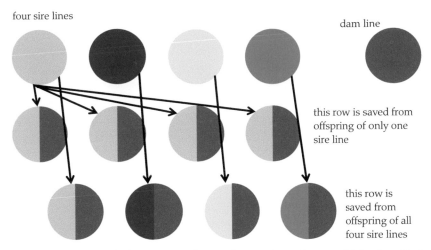

Figure 5.10 Consequences of selecting sons from only one sire or from multiple sires. Each generation is one half the sire's line and one half the dam's line. Using sires from only one line constrains future generations to all have that half in common. Figure by DPS.

a major logistical headache because of its widespread influence throughout the breed. A much more secure path is to make slow progress by making certain that no single animal becomes over-represented in a breed.

5.11 Balancing Bloodlines

Most breeds have multiple bloodlines within them. In some breeds this can involve fairly extreme differences, such as the show lines and field trial lines of several breeds. Even within these divisions, though, most breeds have multiple bloodlines. The management of these bloodlines over time is a delicate endeavor.

It is very tempting for many or most breeders to go back to a single source for any outside breeding. This is usually a highly successful line. Success depends on a host of factors, including genetic potential, but also the ability of the manager to bring that potential to full flower. The "genetic potential" piece implies that a very few sources might indeed actually be superior to all others. Many dog breeders adopt this idea and pursue dogs from these elite kennels. The problem with this approach is that it focuses on individual dogs rather than the breed as a whole. When breeds are viewed as a "whole" it becomes more obvious that it is wise to keep various components in play so that these can be separated out and recombined as desired over the long term. From a genetic management point of view, some level of variation and diversity is highly advantageous in its own right. This can unfortunately occur at some expense to dedicated breeders but is necessary for long-term breed genetic health.

This leads to the conclusion that managing bloodlines within a breed is important. This is more an issue of ensuring that different bloodlines are maintained, rather than what those specific bloodlines should be. To maintain distinctions among bloodlines it is wisest to have at least some breeders maintaining a bloodline in relative isolation from the rest of the breed. Rare bloodlines, for example, disappear completely if they are mated back into common bloodlines. In the process they lose their genetic distinctiveness. This is not to imply that a dog of a rare bloodline should never be mated to a dog of a common bloodline. It is, however, wise to assure that several matings are "rare bloodline" to "rare bloodline" to assure that not all genetic variation is swallowed up into the common bloodlines. They can swamp the rare bloodlines if not managed wisely (Figure 5.11).

There are also hazards on the opposite end of the spectrum. If rarity in and of itself becomes the target of selection and promotion, this can easily lead to some odd dynamics in population genetics. While selection targeted only at performance potential can lead to a poor population structure, the opposite situation of attention to population structure at the expense of other factors can lead to declines in performance potential. As with most selection, a balance of factors is important to achieve overall and long-lasting success.

Some examples of a push for rarity include various fads based on color or other somewhat trivial physical traits that do not closely relate to either performance potential or to population structure. Fads based on traits such as color are highly likely to sample a genetic pool only minimally, which necessarily leads to inbreeding and the dangers that it imposes over the long term.

5.12 Sound Strategies Lead to Sound Breeds

Behind any concern for breed management needs to be an appreciation for what breeds are and why they are useful. Their usefulness comes mostly from their predictability, across all traits both physical and mental. Predictability comes from that unique combination of foundation, isolation, and selection that characterizes every breed. When any of these three becomes extreme, absolute, and inviolable, any one of them can actually provide for weakness instead of strength in breed management.

Foundation, as an example, serves well to set out the original limits of a breed. Most breeds originated from somewhat local dogs at some point in the past, and that sort of foundation is largely gone in most regions. However, it does persist in some breeds. The Basenji, for example, still occurs as a large population of village dogs in portions of Africa. From that large population, a subset was then taken to Europe and the USA to become

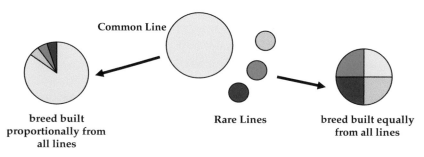

Figure 5.11 Bloodlines can be managed so that the descendant breed can take advantage of all of them and not just the most popular one. Figure by DPS.

what is the Basenji in most kennel clubs. This is essentially a "sub foundation" and exactly how that more restricted sample relates back to the original location is an important issue.

The most important point is that the dogs in Africa are just as much "Basenji" as the dogs outside of Africa, and indeed could be considered to be more so. The point here is that the non-African portions of the breed have a unique situation where they can go back to the original source to refresh and renew the genetic variation in their breed. This heavily depends on registry rules, but ideally, they reflect the concept that nearly all breeds pre-date registries, rather than being created by them. This is a subtle point and is especially true of local and indigenous breeds.

The luxury of repeatedly going back to an original source is not available for many other breeds because the original foundation is long gone. Even for these breeds, though, other breeds are usually available that are closely related by either history, geography, breeding, or purpose. When such cousin breeds are available it can be wise in some specific situations to provide for inclusion of a few dogs that result from outcrosses. This is best done openly and honestly rather than fraudulently. Remember, the goal is predictability, and this can be easily lost if non-typical dogs with very divergent genetics are brought into a breed.

The details of any inclusion of a breeding dog from outside a breed vary widely from breed to breed, and breed group to breed group. Some breeds within a group are fairly closely related by foundation and history, as well as by current type and ability. Coonhounds (other than Blue Tick) generally fall into this sort of group. It could be argued that Retrievers fit into a reasonably closely related group, and Setters into another. The same is true of other breed groups. In contrast, some breed groups contain breeds that are more divergent. In that situation, more caution is warranted in going outside of any one breed.

In some instances, an outcross is needed to correct a specific problem. This has recently been done with the Dalmatian to correct a metabolic peculiarity of metabolism related to urinary stone formation. Such a strategy needs to walk a tightrope between changing the breed or its function on the one hand and providing no change to the metabolism on the other. This is a difficult balancing act, and breeders need to educate themselves about the hazards and the strategies for circumventing them.

Solving genetic problems based on including new dogs into a breed's foundation is a potential strategy but is counter to the "isolation" piece of breed development and which is also important to breed character and function. Immediate acceptance of a dog from another breed into a recipient breed is too drastic in nearly every situation. Similarly, inclusion of a "first-cross" dog would still be a high risk, depending on the goals. Somewhere in the second or third generation of a backcross to the original breed, though, is likely a spot where the genetic problem has been corrected and the original breed's predictability is high enough to serve well in its role.

Selection, the third basis of breed formation, is ongoing and is a powerful tool for either causing or solving problems. When breeders formulate goals that work for long-term soundness and serviceability of dogs, the result is that the dogs, the dog breeders, and the dog breed all benefit. When more short-term goals are desired, problems can arise. This is especially true when extremes are the goal of selection. Extremes can lead to unsoundness, and this has implications for the establishment of wise goals and approaches.

Unfortunately, the single most useful trait for selecting soundness is longevity. Dogs that remain healthy through a long life have escaped major diseases and have also presented few enough management problems so that they were not eliminated for that reason. For a host of reasons this is an unrealistic selection target in dogs, because fertility drops off with age and females must be managed for earlier reproduction rather than for very late repro-duction. Still, there are various conformational predictors of success in longevity, and these should be used whenever possible. Some selection goals, such as free-whelping in several of the short-headed breeds, could be easily instituted and would quickly change the overall type and soundness of the breed. Obviously, these would have to be embraced rather than shunned by the breeders, judges, and customers interested in puppies. Ultimately it is market demand that is going to determine the most popular model of dog within each breed. This is where short-term pressures may well be contrary to long-term welfare.

5.13 Designer Dogs and Crossbreds

A few thoughts are warranted concerning a recent trend for crossing specific breeds to produce what can be called "designer dogs." Sometimes these are referred to as "designer breeds," but they lack the important aspect of genetic isolation and genetic uniformity that characterizes true genetic breeds (Figure 5.12). These attempts usually strive to achieve a balance between the desired traits of both breeds. The mating of Labrador Retrievers and

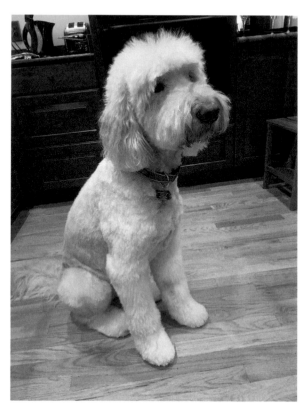

Figure 5.12 Goldendoodles are a cross between Golden Retrievers and Poodles and have become highly appreciated by their owners. Photo by Paula Stith.

Poodles to produce Labradoodles is one such example among an ever-increasing array of these named hybrids.

This strategy has several interesting aspects. One very real advantage is that it brings hybrid vigor to the puppies. They can be expected, on average, to be much more heterozygous and therefore somewhat more robust than purebreds. This varies enough that the rule should not be considered absolute, but it still holds true on average. This does not mean that such dogs are completely free of all risk, although many breeders of these dogs do promote this faulty assumption, and many buyers willingly accept it as true.

A second advantage for crossbreds springs from the fact that most breeds do not widely share identical defective alleles for genetic diseases that are controlled by single alleles. Again, there are many exceptions to this rule, especially for polygenic traits such as hip dysplasia. However, it is generally true that crossing breeds diminishes the chances of producing a homozygote for a genetic disease caused by a single allele.

Any success of crossbreeding very much depends on viable and available pure breeds. While the first crossbred offspring are fairly narrowly predictable, those crossbred animals are themselves very unpredictable in what they will produce. For example, a mating between two Labradoodles can result in puppies that resemble Labradors, puppies that resemble Poodles, and everything in between, including new combinations that might not be obvious and that deviate not only from the two parental breeds, but also from that first cross. What this means is that the strategy of crossbreeding can be productive in that first cross, but then hits a dead-end where predictability declines in succeeding generations. While selection can be imposed to narrow the variation down to the desired blend of the two foundation breeds, this is inherently wasteful because only a few puppies will have the desired combination.

The trajectory of the genetic consequences of a strategy that takes crossbreeding through several generations therefore indicates that the first cross is reasonably predictable, but this strategy abruptly ceases to be constructive if it goes beyond that first crossbred generation. Even under the assumption that crossbreeding is a useful strategy in some rare instances, it always depends on the availability of pure breeds. Crossbred dogs have essentially no constructive role to play in the production of future generations. Therefore, even though some breeders may resort to crossbreeding, this strategy still depends on maintenance of distinct breeds as predictable and useful genetic resources.

5.14 Key Points

- Genetic management of dog breeds assures their survival as useful genetic resources that are predictable for final appearance and function.
- Effective management is holistic and relies on more than a handful of easy details.
- Strong breeds can be achieved by balancing linebreeding and linecrossing.
- Coefficients of inbreeding and kinship measurements can be useful tools but need to be used wisely.
- Crossbreeding "uses up" genetic material while not contributing to its continuation in predictable genetic pools.

CHAPTER 6

General Health Management

6.1 Routine Care

Routine veterinary wellness care is important for all dogs, and especially for breeding animals because they need to be healthy to support reproduction. Any change in the systemic health status of either males or females can affect fertility and the breeding program. A brood bitch needs to be healthy to cycle normally, become pregnant, carry the pregnancy to term, and raise her puppies. A male breeding dog needs to maintain general health to be able to produce normal sperm cells in adequate numbers for a successful mating and the conception of a litter.

Annual health screening is a useful tool in monitoring health, but the details for various diseases vary from region to region. Throughout most of the USA, screening for heartworm and tick-borne diseases is recommended. These diseases are increasingly widespread and potentially have a negative effect on fertility. The best way to prevent many severe diseases is vaccination, and this is even more important when dogs are housed together in kennels, encounter one another in competitive events, or are brought together for mating. Breeding stock should always be up to date on core vaccinations, and on any optional vaccinations that are appropriate for the specific lifestyles or activities of the dog.

6.2 Vaccines, Preventatives, and Therapeutic Drugs

Vaccines for dogs are now widely available and new ones are constantly being introduced. Whether or not an individual dog needs a specific vaccine depends on the overall likelihood of encountering the disease, as well as the severity of the disease should it occur. Vaccination of breeding females is especially important regardless of her own risk of encountering various disease agents, because when she is well-vaccinated, she can pass protection along to her puppies.

Vaccines can be broken down into various groups.

- Core vaccines are those that protect against disease agents that produce serious diseases and are likely to be encountered by most dogs. Many of these are included in combination vaccines that protect for several different agents:
  o distemper virus
  o parvovirus
  o parainfluenza virus
  o adenovirus
  o rabies (except in countries where the disease does not occur).
- Lifestyle vaccines are those that depend on an individual dog's risk of exposure. Dogs that are routinely exposed to other dogs or to livestock are recommended to have most of these:
  o *Bordetella*
  o canine influenza
  o leptospirosis
  o Lyme disease.

In most regions, all dogs should be on some form of year-round heartworm and internal parasite prevention regime. Many products are currently available for these needs, but the specific product for use in breeding dogs needs to be carefully selected because a few of them are not safe for use in breeding animals. It is important that the package inserts are studied carefully and that breeders are familiar with the active ingredients in products used for routine parasite prevention as several of them are not recommended for use in breeding dogs.

Fortunately, research on many products has proved that they do not impair reproduction and their use is known to be safe in breeding animals. Current recommendations include the following drug classes for heartworm prevention as well as flea and tick prevention:

- ivermectin
- milbemycin
- selamectin
- fipronil
- (s)Methoprene
- imidacloprid
- Flumethrin.

Isoxazoline-substituted benzamide derivatives have had adverse results in safety studies and should be avoided:

- spinosad
- afoxolaner
- sarolaner
- fluralaner.

Not all pharmaceuticals are benign to breeding stock, and unfortunately the entire list is constantly changing as studies and experience advance. Several products, including several antibiotics, are detrimental to semen production. Several products are documented as causing abnormalities in developing embryos. The use of any drug in breeding stock should be considered only with veterinary consultation, and preferably by a veterinarian certified or especially interested in canine reproduction. Use of any drug requires careful consideration of the level of risk compared to the anticipated level of benefit. All breeders should read product inserts very carefully before they discuss the use of a pharmaceutical with their veterinarian. This is especially the case for a dog that is actively breeding or that has been mated and is pregnant.

Some breeders have adopted an unfortunate strategy of routinely using therapeutic products, including antibiotics, even in the absence of any specific documented need. This strategy should be actively avoided. Using any product in the absence of a real need for it runs a risk of a negative outcome, including any direct adverse or toxic effects on reproduction. Routine use also facilitates the development of resistance to the product by its target, resulting in a reduction of the effectiveness of the product in situations when it is truly needed to combat a specific problem. This is an especially common outcome to the unrestricted use of antibiotics and has led to the development of antibiotic resistance in some bacteria.

6.3 Diets and Feeding

Diet influences the overall health of animals and their ability to exercise and maintain a proper body condition. The gastrointestinal tract of the domesticated dog has important differences from that of its wolf ancestors. Dogs are domesticated animals and, while they descend from wolves, they have many important and consistent changes from their wolf ancestors. A major change that domestication produced is the ability of dogs to use a wider variety of feed sources than would sustain a wolf.

Dogs digest carbohydrates (starches) much more easily and completely than wolves do and are therefore able to get more nutrient value from grain sources than wolves can. Commercial canine diets are formulated with this important difference in mind and are targeted for the gastrointestinal digestive abilities of modern dogs. Commercial diets are an appropriate choice in nearly all situations because they reflect the specific nutritional needs of dogs and appropriately support both growth and maintenance.

Appropriate diets for breeding stock are essential. Breeding dogs should be in good body condition before any reproduction occurs. An appropriate plane of nutrition contributes to this. Excess weight in female dogs is detrimental to normal estrus cyclicity, ovulation rates, pregnancy, and whelping. Overly fat male dogs can accumulate fat within the scrotum. This leads to an increase in temperature of the testes and poor spermatogenesis.

When seen from the side, dogs with an ideal weight have an abdominal tuck up from the bottomline and a narrowing at the waist that can be viewed looking down from above. The ribs should be easily felt, although not easily counted from afar. In most cases, if someone has to ask if their dog is overweight, the answer is likely "yes." Dogs that are overweight are much more common than those that are in an appropriate, or even a thin, body condition. Obesity has negative effects on fertility and shortens the dog's life span.

A balanced commercial diet is appropriate for dogs in most situations. Commercial diets are labeled for the specific types of dogs and life stages that they are designed to serve.

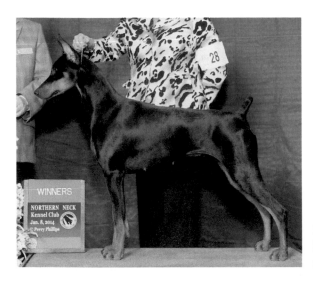

Figure 6.1 Dogs in ideal condition are fit, lean, and have an obvious "tuck" in the abdomen. Photo by Beverly Purswell.

Those labeled for "growth and reproduction" or for "all life stages" are appropriate for nearly all dogs. These labels indicate that the diet is adequate for pregnancy, lactation, and puppy growth. The label means that the diet is certified as meeting the ingredient standards of the Association of American Feed Control Officials (AAFCO), or that the manufacturer has provided results of a feeding trial that satisfies AAFCO standards. Current recommendations for all dogs in a breeding program include maintaining them all on a balanced, commercial dog food.

Abrupt or frequent changes in diet negatively affect the ability of dogs to digest their food and absorb appropriate nutrients. Changes also risk the alteration of normal gastrointestinal microflora that is made up of beneficial bacteria and other small organisms. These changes can lead to dysbiosis, which is a change in the microflora that resides in the gut. The result is gastrointestinal upset.

Adding any supplements to an appropriately formulated diet risks unbalancing the diet. Currently there is no firm evidence that demonstrates that any specific supplement increases fecundity (litter size) of the males or females fed the supplement. Many supplements contain ingredients that are known to be detrimental to fertility, and so these should be used cautiously, if at all.

Feeding "boutique" diets should only be done with great caution. These diets have more frequent recalls when compared to major brands. Recalls are generally due to contamination with infectious agents or chemicals, or for some other significant problem with the diet. These can adversely affect dog health and reproduction. Some of these diets have led to an increase in the rate of cardiac defects in animals fed with the diet. Diets from major brands are much less likely to cause any illness than are boutique diets and have more adequate scientific data supporting any dietary claim.

Raw diets are not recommended. Abortion and neonatal death have been linked to contamination by *Salmonella spp.* and *Campylobacter spp.* coming from raw diets. Both bacteria have been implicated in severe systemic infections, which in some cases has resulted in death of dogs. Raw diets often have variable vitamin and mineral content, and these might not always adequately meet nutritional needs of a breeding animal. There are no scientifically proven benefits of a raw diet when compared to a commercial or cooked diet.

Some owners continue to prefer to cook for their animals despite the availability of reliable commercial diets. In this situation the final diet needs to be well-balanced. This nearly always requires the aid of a veterinary nutritionist. Home-prepared diets will generally require the addition of micro- and macronutrients obtained from a trusted veterinary source. A balanced diet is essential. Failing to meet the nutritional needs of breeding dogs will negatively impact their ability to maintain systemic health and fertility.

6.4 *Exercise and Social Stimulation*

Exercise and environmental enrichment are essential for breeding stock. Daily exercise should be a part of any animal's routine. There are many exercise options for a busy kennel or a small breeding operation. Treadmills, both self-propelled as well as motor driven, are available. "Roading" animals with a golf cart or 4-wheeler is another good option to exercise groups dogs. A minimum of about 30 minutes of aerobic exercise is needed every day, although higher amounts are generally preferable.

Exercising animals not only increases their aerobic and anaerobic capacity, but also increases muscle mass and decreases excess fat deposition. Exercise is also a great form of enrichment and stimulation for dogs. Dogs are curious by nature and easily become bored without some sort of stimulation. Getting dogs active on a daily basis provides mental stimulation and decreases stereotypies or other undesirable behaviors.

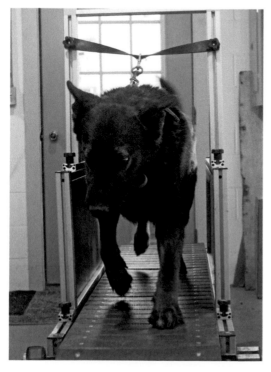

Figure 6.2 This dog is being kept in good physical condition by exercising on a treadmill. Photo by Jill Keaton.

Daily interaction between managers or owners and dogs allows for training opportunities and socialization. Basic obedience training is a good baseline for all dogs. Training to advanced levels in obedience, hunting, agility, or other activities are all highly recommended, with the specific activity based on the natural instincts bred into the specific breed of dog. A kennel that is good at routine training and socialization activities will be well prepared for these same essential activities when puppies arrive. Puppies require stimulation and socialization during their young lives, because this primes them for a rich and successful life of partnership with their owners.

6.5 Biosecurity

Biosecurity is often overlooked but is very important in all parts of the breeding cycle from mating to whelping, through to the early life of the puppies. Biosecurity in the last three weeks of the pregnant bitch's gestation and the first three weeks after whelping are especially important. This is known as the "six-week rule." A few practices need to be in place prior to this six-week period that drastically reduce or eliminate the possibility of any dog-to-dog transfer of infectious diseases to the dam or to the puppies.

One good biosecurity practice is to be sure to follow a specific order when caring for the dogs within the kennel. The recommended order is based on the degree of immuno-compromise within the various age groups and types of dogs in the kennel. Best practice involves feeding, managing, and treating dogs starting with the most vulnerable first and ending with the least vulnerable. An example of a good sequence to use, from most to least vulnerable, is:

1 bitches that have puppies younger than three weeks old
2 bitches that have puppies over three weeks old
3 pregnant bitches
4 permanent resident dogs that do not travel outside of the kennel.

Two groups of dogs should ideally be separated from the first four, and from each other, by a physical quarantine barrier:

5 dogs from the kennel that are actively travelling to shows or events
6 new arrivals that are under quarantine.

Caretakers should change clothes and wash their hands when an animal in one of the earlier groups needs to be cared for after working with animals in one of the later care levels. This is especially true if they have been handling dogs that have been travelling. The goal is to eliminate any risk of infection prior to handling any pregnant bitches or bitches with puppies.

No new dogs, or traveling dogs, should be introduced into the kennel without a strict four-week (or longer) quarantine period. This length of time allows for any disease(s) to which the dog may have been exposed to become outwardly apparent prior to them being introduced to the general population of the kennel.

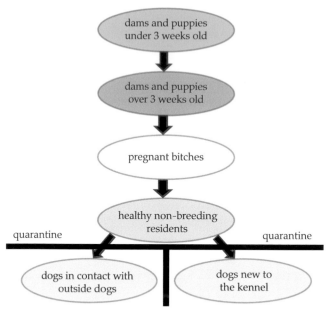

Figure 6.3 A good sequence of caring for the various sorts of dogs within a kennel works to protect the most vulnerable members of the kennel. Dogs that are new to the kennel should be quarantined separately from the dogs of the kennel that have contact with outside dogs. Figure by JTC.

Owners should always be cautious as to how many people interact with the bitch and her puppies during the first few weeks of life. Humans can easily mechanically transfer diseases from dog to dog simply from surface contamination. Visitors should wear clean clothing, wash their hands prior to handling puppies or the dam, and remove their shoes before entering the kennel area. Stricter measures with bleach foot baths and outer protective clothing can be used but are usually not necessary in small breeding operations. These procedures considerably reduce the chance of disease transfer to the pregnant bitch and her puppies.

6.6 Key Points

- Dogs used for breeding benefit from good routine management.
- Vaccination protocols are important to limit disease.
- Vaccination is especially important for dogs that are campaigned or that travel for mating.
- Routine parasite control is an important baseline for health.
- Diets for breeding dogs need to be well-balanced.
- Many "fad diets" are not balanced and are difficult to balance.
- Obesity should always be avoided in breeding dogs.
- Dogs used for breeding benefit from exercise.
- Dogs used for breeding benefit from socialization and social stimulation.
- Biosecurity keeps the dam and her puppies as safe as possible.
- Dogs should be cared for in a sequence that protects each one.
- Dogs that travel or are newly introduced should be quarantined away from resident dogs.

CHAPTER 7

Management of the Male

The contribution of the male dog is often taken for granted, and it must be emphasized that the male dog contributes an important fifty percent to the genetics of any litter he sires. His fertility is essential to produce a viable and healthy litter, and any lack of male fertility has total veto over the outcome of a mating. Male breeding dogs need to be in good health to produce normal sperm cells in sufficient numbers to conceive a litter. In addition to general health and well-being, other important factors include:

- diet
- exercise
- reproductive tract health
- routine breeding soundness examinations for male dogs that are actively used for breeding.

Male dogs tend to be the ones most often blamed for any failure of reproduction. Owners of a breeding male can be sure that they are holding up their end of the bargain by ensuring that their male is healthy, able to breed, and able to produce puppies. Owners should take the time to become educated to provide the best quality product possible and should be prepared to adjust if problems arise.

Knowing the basics about how sperm cells are produced aids the understanding of the many factors that affect the fertility of a male dog. The production of fertile mature sperm is called spermatogenesis. It depends on an intricate cycle of cell division and maturation within the seminiferous tubules of the testes. The entire cellular cycle from a sperm precursor to a fully developed sperm cell takes approximately 62 days (Figure 7.1). It is important to keep this period in mind when considering any problems that can arise in sperm quality and fertility. Due to the time lag inherent in the 62 day cycle, there is a delay from the initial damage to its final result in abnormal mature sperm. This time lag influences the need for and the schedule followed for recheck appointments when any high profile matings are planned after adverse health events, especially those that result in elevated body temperature or severe alterations of basic physiologic processes. Any elevated fever in a male

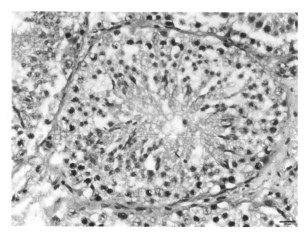

Figure 7.1 Sperm are produced by the cells lining the tubules in the testes. The cells go through a series of cell divisions and other processes of maturation as they progress from the base of the tubule and move into its center. At that point they are mature sperm and are passed along to the next portion of the male reproductive tract to be available for fertilization. The entire process with the sperm cell moving from the base of the tubule to its center takes about 62 days. Photo by T.E. Cecere.

breeding dog negatively affects sperm formation, which may take two months to become evident. Fever can also have direct and immediate negative consequences for sperm that are already mature. Poor semen quality can persist for at least two months after the illness has abated.

In addition to the influences imposed by the biological underpinnings of sperm production, are various factors that arise from the management of breeding dogs. Owners of male breeding dogs are under pressure to provide breeding services from their male in a timely manner. Those services need to produce results in the form of vigorous puppies. Preparing to stand a male dog at stud involves considering both the physiology of reproduction and business arrangements. Contracts describing the services offered are always recommended. This ensures that both parties are aware of the terms of service and what the expected outcomes are for that service. Many a male dog has been blamed for failure to conceive a litter, even when the failure may have not been the male's fault. Contracts can help to dispel any future disagreements. Terms of the contract can include the type of mating, timing, method, and location of that mating, payment plans for the stud fee(s), and what happens in the event of a failure to conceive a litter. These terms should be clear and provided in written form. Legal counsel should be consulted to make sure that any written contract is valid and legally binding.

7.1 *Male Growth and Development*

Basic growth and development of the male dog are important baselines to consider for breeding animals. Puppies are born with all of their major organs already formed. Many organs are functional at birth, others are not fully functional but are ready to begin their final growth, to undergo final maturation at an appropriate age. From about 8 weeks and up to the age of puberty, the body concentrates on growth and behavioral development. The male reproductive organs grow during this period, but only achieve their final maturation to fertility beginning at puberty.

Puppies reach puberty at various ages depending on breed and final adult body size. Puberty usually occurs when dogs reach a growth plateau where growth slows from the

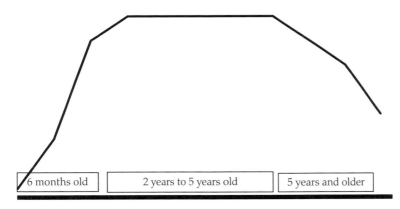

Figure 7.2 The fertility of male dogs usually begins to rise quickly at about 6 months old, reaches a peak at about 2 years, and then begins to fall off after 5 years or so. Figure by DPS.

rapid rate earlier in life. At this point, the testes begin producing testosterone and sperm cells. This happens at around six months old for most dogs and across most breeds. Many dogs are fertile at this early age, although most males require another 12 to 18 months to produce the full complement of normal sperm cells in high enough numbers to be fully fertile (Figure 7.2). Male dogs therefore come into full fertility fairly slowly. At the other end of life, fertility declines as age advances. Maximum fertility in most male dogs is between about two years and six years old, preceded by a gradual rise and then followed by a gradual decline.

Even though the final mature reproductive tract takes time to develop, a few potential problems are obvious even at relatively early ages. Cryptorchidism is the failure of the testes to fully descend into the scrotum. Cryptorchid puppies can generally be identified at a young age and although opinions on this vary, this identification should ideally occur at the breeder's home prior to the puppy being sold. Both testes should be descended into the scrotum prior to three months of age. Some references state that full descent can take up to six months to occur, but this somewhat delayed period comes with a note of caution. Many family lines with delayed testicular descent have gone on to experience reduced fertility and fully cryptorchid males a few generations after delayed testicular descent was first noticed in males of the bloodline. This risk of increasingly severe problems over sequential generations is not uniform across all lines but is generally a risk not worth taking. Breeders that are working to improve a bloodline should avoid males with slow or incomplete descent of testes. Ignoring the problem of delayed descent can lead to a bloodline that begins to produce cryptorchid puppies, and at that point there is no easy solution to the problem.

7.2 Nutrition of the Male Dog

Male dogs are most easily supported by feeding balanced commercial diets labeled as suitable for "all life stages." Dietary supplements have not been definitively proven to support spermatogenesis or to improve overall sperm quality or numbers. If supplements are provided, prudent owners should carefully read every label and know the ingredients in each one. Nutraceuticals, and this includes most supplements, are not regulated by the Food and Drug Administration (FDA) of the USA. Many of them have unsubstantiated claims of quality, and this can even include the actual amounts of each ingredient. Aside from the generally vague quality or potential contribution of most supplements, many feed stuffs have been proven to have a detrimental effect on sperm quality or numbers. Caution is warranted when using these.

The list of dietary supplements that are known to be safe and possibly helpful for the male breeding dog, is very short. These have been found to possibly have a positive effect on the male dog's semen evaluation. However, these should only be supplemented with the advice of a veterinarian and sourced from a veterinary provider. Supplements with potential positive effects include:

- fatty acid supplements (fish oil)
- vitamin E
- selenium
- zinc
- glucosamine and glycosaminoglycans
- carnitine.

Some of these supplements, when given in excessive amounts, then become detrimental instead of helpful. Supplements must therefore be used cautiously, with an understanding that their use can alter the balanced diet that is already being fed. Glucosamine and fish oil supplements are generally safe to add to a male dog's feeding routine but are only recommended if the diet does not already contain adequate amounts.

A few supplements have been proven to be detrimental and should be avoided, even in small amounts. If a supplement falls within one of these categories, the safety studies should be evaluated before their use. The supplements to avoid include:

- cottonseed meal (contains gossypol)
- estrogenic compounds
- some specific antibiotics, antifungals, anti-inflammatory and other drugs (currently there are approximately 45 drugs that have been shown to have detrimental effects on spermatogenesis in the dog)
- some specific heartworm preventatives (covered in Chapter 6)
- some specific flea and tick products (covered in Chapter 6).

Owners of actively breeding male dogs should work closely with a veterinarian to be sure that the dog is only being prescribed products for which the benefit clearly outweighs the risk of negatively affecting sperm quality. It is best to closely read product labels for anything being considered for either supplementation or a treatment for a medical condition. Paying close attention to detail assures that an informed decision can be made on the use of any product. Peer-reviewed literature is the best source for knowing what to feed and what to avoid, and prudent breeders make sure to read the literature firsthand so that they can be confident that what they are feeding is benefiting the dog and not harming him.

7.3 *Exercise and Fitness*

Male breeding dogs require a healthy body condition to maintain normal spermatogenesis. This includes not only appropriate nutrition, but also exercise (Figure 7.3). Lasting effects on a dog's ability to produce normal sperm cells can result from either too much exercise, or too little.

Normal spermatogenesis occurs in the scrotum a few degrees cooler than normal body temperature, about 3–5°F (1.5–2.5°C). Any situation that raises the body temperature above normal carries the possibility of damaging the sperm cells within the testis and impairing the ability of the testis to carry out normal spermatogenesis. Heavy exercise can elevate the scrotal temperature out of the normal range, although the actual rise in temperature depends on the conditioning of the individual dog and its history of exercise. A dog in heavy training in hot weather is a recipe for disaster because the cooler scrotal temperature becomes impossible to maintain. While it is most ideal to completely avoid these temperature rises, dogs used for performance or work cannot always avoid the conditions that lead to excess heat. In those situations, keeping the animal out in the heat for as little time as possible and getting them back into a cool environment as quickly as possible is key to minimizing any adverse effect on spermatogenesis.

Schedules for mating a male dog should consider any previous hot sporting events or show schedules that a male dog may have undergone during the previous 62 days. This is a consequence of the time lag between a precursor cell being affected by a single day of hot competition and the final functional sperm that is produced from that precursor. This time lag requires owners to think forward two months to warn the owners of potential mates about the potential of reduced fertility. It generally takes about 10 days after a heat insult to see negative effects on the sperm cells, and these effects can then persist for nearly 50 more days. A breeding soundness examination within a week of a potential mate coming into estrus helps to alleviate any concerns over the fertility of the male.

Some sources of excess heat are not particularly obvious but can still cause significant damage. Heavily coated breeds are often prepared for the show ring by hot blow drying

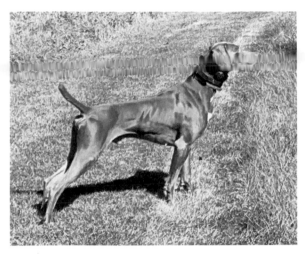

Figure 7.3 Fit males are more able to mate and conceive a litter than are less athletic males. This Weimaraner is in extremely fit body condition and is also demonstrating ability appropriate for the breed. Photo by Meredith Wadsworth.

the coat. This can raise body temperature sufficiently to negatively affect their sperm-making capacity. Using forced (not hot) air is much preferred to hot air blow drying. Avoiding hot air reduces the number of sperm abnormalities that are related to heat damage.

Male dogs that are overweight or obese encounter multiple challenges that can result in elevated temperatures. Overweight males must work harder at exercise due to the excess fat that the dog carries. As a result, their body temperature increases faster than that of a leaner dog. This is due to the excess fat that the dog carries. Fat provides a layer of insulation, and male dogs store excess fat within the scrotum. This extra insulation impairs the scrotum's natural ability to lose heat into the environment and results in higher temperatures, which can be sufficiently high that they diminish spermatogenesis. Keeping male dogs lean is a general recommendation to avoid impaired fertility due to heat-related sperm damage. Although it is important to exercise the dog frequently to curb any excess fat storage, it is equally important that hot events are avoided, and time spent working in the heat is limited.

7.4 *Prostate Health*

The prostate gland is the only accessory sex gland in the male dog. This gland is contained within the pelvic canal and surrounds the urethra. It serves as the main source of fluid in an ejaculate and contributes to creating the hydrostatic pressure that forces sperm cells through the cervix of a bitch during a natural mating. Two common conditions of the prostate gland that are of concern with an actively breeding male are:

- benign prostatic hyperplasia (BPH)
- prostatitis (inflammation of the prostate gland).

The prostate is responsive to blood levels of testosterone and its active counterpart, dihydrotestosterone (DHT). The amount of testosterone increases as males age beyond puberty, which causes the prostate to enlarge to its adult size. In some males this normal change can continue beyond a size that is normal for an intact male. This excess growth is most likely to occur during or after middle age. An excessive growth of the prostate is called benign prostatic hyperplasia (BPH). Not all males with an enlarged prostate will have clinical signs, which may include difficulty in urination or defecation. The age of clinical diagnosis is usually about eight years old, with a range of three years in either direction. Some of the affected males have blood in their ejaculate or urine. A full examination is warranted if the prostate is enlarged or painful on examination, if blood is noted in collected semen, or if blood is present when voiding urine.

Blood in prostatic fluid presents two problems (Figure 7.4). It is directly damaging to sperm, and it is also a very good bacterial culture medium. When blood is present in the prostate, bacteria can easily overgrow and cause a clinically important inflammatory process. The result of this would be prostatitis from a secondary bacterial infection of the prostate. Affected animals are sometimes febrile and may also have signs associated with pain or difficulty urinating or defecating.

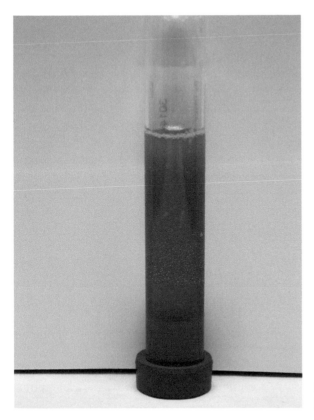

Figure 7.4 Bloody or discolored prostatic fluid is a sign of prostatitis. Photo by JTC.

Benign prostatic hyperplasia should be treated before it becomes prostatitis, which is fortunately easy to accomplish. The first step is a veterinary examination which includes diagnostic procedures and tests. This can document the presence of benign prostatic hyperplasia, which can then be treated with one of the drugs that reduces the conversion of testosterone to dihydrotestosterone. Therapy for benign prostatic hyperplasia generally lasts six to eight weeks, and it is common to have recheck evaluations after completion of treatment. Some males are more prone to clinical signs accompanying benign prostatic hyperplasia than are others, so management is best tailored on a case-by-case basis. Persistent benign prostatic hyperplasia is easily controlled with periodic administration of one of the drugs. Frequent rechecks under veterinary supervision will help to manage the situation. Once a male dog is finished with its breeding career, castration can permanently cure benign prostatic hyperplasia.

Animals with active prostatitis are usually treated for six to eight weeks with both an antibiotic and a drug that reduces dihydrotestosterone levels. Some specific antibiotics are effective, and others are not. This is due to the blood-prostate barrier that prevents absorption of some antibiotics. Early and accurate diagnosis and treatment of both benign prostatic hyperplasia and prostatitis will eliminate several potential problems during a male dog's breeding career.

The testes can also be the source of problems for male dogs. The most common conditions are testicular neoplasms (tumors). The most common age of onset is 8 years old.

About 90% of the neoplasms of the reproductive tract of male dogs are testicular tumors. The three most common types of neoplasms are related to the cell types of the testis, and include seminomas, interstitial (Leydig) cell tumors, and Sertoli cell tumors. Most tumors are benign, although they can affect the male's fertility. They are often bilateral, so in cases where a mass is palpated, it is wise to do a thorough examination (including ultrasound) of the opposite testis to document the presence or absence of a mass in it.

Interstitial (Leydig) cell tumors are slightly more common than the others but are usually somewhat silent clinically. They often cause some level of degeneration of the seminiferous tubules, and semen quality can therefore suffer. A favorable outcome for fertility can occur in situations where the degeneration has not progressed very far, and the tumor is in only one testis. In these cases, a hemicastration of only the affected testis can lead to recovery of fertility in the remaining testis. Fertility usually returns to 50% to 60% of the level that was present before the tumor developed.

Sertoli cell tumors are more likely to be clinically evident, because they can produce estrogen which feminizes the male dog. About half of the males with this sort of tumor will have development of the mammary chain, hair loss with hyperpigmentation of the skin, and will also become attractive to other male dogs due to the pheromones they produce. The estrogen production also leads to degeneration of the seminiferous tubules, with a decline in semen quality. When the mass is only present in one testis, hemicastration can return some males to fertility.

Seminomas have less effect on fertility than do the other two types of testicular tumors. Affected testes should be removed, though, to prevent progression to a malignant state that can threaten the dog's life.

Other testicular conditions are rare and include torsion of the testis, and testicular inflammation due to infection. Torsion is sudden and painful, and the only effective treatment is removal of the affected testis. Inflammation of the testis is called "orchitis" and can be secondary to infection by several different organisms. For example, *Brucella canis* is one of the organisms that can be responsible for orchitis, so any dog with orchitis should be tested for brucellosis.

7.5 *Breeding Soundness Examination (BSE)*

Breeding soundness examinations (BSEs) are important and useful tools for managing a male breeding dog. They should be done frequently enough that the owner has consistently good data to be alerted early to any emerging problems. Breeding soundness examinations are necessary because male fertility can change quite rapidly with changing stress levels, environmental alterations, and age. Early changes in fertility are often subject to successful management, while long-term untreated problems can result in permanent impairment.

Breeding soundness examinations should be performed by a veterinarian that has had extra training in semen evaluation to assure the most accurate information possible. A complete breeding soundness examination includes:

- evaluation of libido
- evaluation of penis and prepuce

- collection of a semen sample for examination of:
  - o color and viscosity of the semen collected
  - o motility of the sperm cells
  - o concentration or numbers of sperm cells in the ejaculate
  - o morphology of the sperm cells
  - o viability of the sperm cells (the proportion that are alive)
- complete physical exam with attention to testes and scrotum.

The evaluator that is doing the breeding soundness examination analysis should provide comments on each of these details of the exam. They should be able to discuss numbers of sperm and volume of semen expected in a breeding dose, as well as how to handle the male dog if any potential problems arise. The details of each portion of the exam can help breeders to be aware of what is expected from a breeding soundness examination.

Evaluation of libido should be performed during all collections. Dogs with adequate libido usually respond to manual stimulation by erection and ejaculation. Nearly all males readily respond to the visual presence and scent of a female in estrus. Dogs that are very shy or have a soft demeanor may need the presence of a female in estrus to fully assess libido. Most male dogs will easily obtain an erection in response to pressure applied to the penis and will rapidly produce all three fractions of an ejaculate. Any interruptions or delays in the process of ejaculation should be taken seriously. These warrant evaluation by a veterinarian when they occur. Poor libido in some individual males can be related to musculoskeletal or prostatic problems, or to obese body condition.

During the collection of semen, the penis and prepuce should be evaluated for any abnormalities. This is relatively easily accomplished during the collection of the semen sample. There are a few defects of the penis and prepuce that are known to be heritable. Among these are a persistent frenulum that connects the penis to the prepuce or to another portion of the penis. Another is a prolapse of the urethra out through the tip of the penis (Figure 7.5). Either of these should be noted during an examination and should be followed by discussions around the genetic mechanisms involved and the future breeding career of the male dog being examined.

Some changes in the penis and prepuce are related to transmissible diseases. These include transmissible venereal tumors and vesicular lesions due to herpes virus. These should be noted, and definitive diagnosis and treatment should be initiated under veterinary supervision. Any ulcerations, lacerations, foreign bodies (grass, hair, and so on) can also be found during collection of an ejaculate. These conditions can all be treated appropriately. The ideal result is that no abnormalities are present on the penis or prepuce.

The next evaluations in the breeding soundness examination all involve examination of the semen produced by the male through ejaculation. Collection of the ejaculate is accomplished by putting manual pressure on the base of the penis. This provides for an erection of the penis, and in males with normal libido this progresses to ejaculation. The ejaculate is collected into a flexible plastic bag. The best ejaculates are obtained from male dogs that are calm and confident during the collection.

Male dogs ejaculate in three fractions. The second fraction is the most important because it is the fraction with sperm in it. Most male dogs produce less than 1–5 ml of a combined

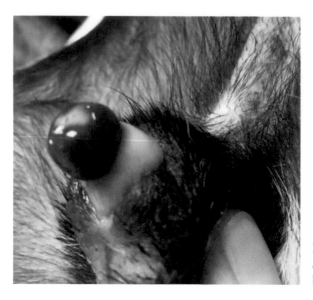

Figure 7.5 Prolapse of the urethra in a male dog is readily observed on a breeding soundness exam. Photo by JTC.

first fraction and second sperm-rich fraction. The third fraction dilutes out the concentration of the first two fractions because it contributes fluid but only very few sperm cells. As a result, a total ejaculate of 15 ml is not necessarily 15 ml of highly concentrated sperm cells because that third fraction has considerably diluted the more valuable second fraction.

The color of the ejaculate should be noted. Deviations from a pale opaque ejaculate are important and can indicate further problems (Figure 7.6).

Sperm motility should be evaluated after the collection has occurred. A pre-warmed glass slide is essential to avoid any cold shock to the cells. The slide is evaluated using a

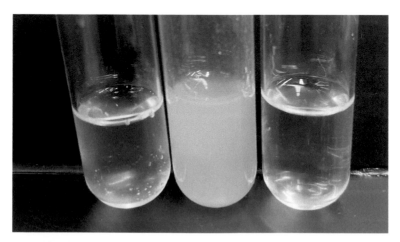

Figure 7.6 The normal dog ejaculate has three fractions. The first fraction contains very few sperm, and the third contains few or none. In this ejaculate the first is contaminated with urine which gives it a slight yellow tinge. It should be possible to read text through samples of the first and third fractions. The second fraction is the sperm-rich fraction and is an opaque white due to the sperm it contains. Photo by JTC.

microscope that allows observation of the cells and their movement. The important aspects in motility include:

- gross motility, or the total proportion of sperm cells that are moving
- progressive motility, which is the proportion of the sperm moving forward in a linear fashion.

Motility evaluation is drastically improved when accomplished by a computer assisted sperm analysis (CASA) machine, although a well-trained individual operator is usually within 5–10% of this machine. It is important to not discount the accuracy of motility scores reported by a trained individual using only a light microscope, because they can have equal accuracy with less expense. Good gross motility should be 70% or higher. If sperm cells are not moving in a linear fashion (for example if they are spinning in circles) this should be noted. Sperm cells will sometimes agglutinate, or stick together, which should also be noted.

Concentration is given as the number of sperm cells within a given volume of the ejaculate. This should ideally be evaluated using either a hemocytometer or a flow cytometry machine. These two methods are both accurate enough to determine the number of sperm cells within an ejaculate. This is an important measurement because the volume of a dog's ejaculate does not correlate well to the actual concentration of sperm. A healthy male should be able to produce 20 million sperm cells per kilogram of body weight, or more than 300 million sperm cells in a single ejaculation. This number can decrease if the animal is being over-used by either mating multiple females in short succession or is having semen collections performed too often. The ideal time interval between collections is 2–3 days.

A low concentration of sperm is known as oligospermia, and the causes include:

- failure to obtain a complete collection
- the animal having a pathologic condition causing low sperm numbers
- the animal has ejaculated the sperm cells into the urinary system.

Regardless of the cause of oligospermia, additional tests can be performed on the fluid obtained during a collection to determine if a full ejaculate was obtained. This can lead the veterinarian to recommend further diagnostics to pinpoint any problems.

Sperm morphology is the physical appearance of individual sperm cells (Figure 7.7). Morphology is evaluated by staining the sperm on a warm slide with a live-dead stain. One commonly used stain is Hancock's stain, also called Eosin-Nigrosin stain. Evaluation of morphology should be performed by a person and not by a machine. A trained individual can identify subtle changes in the sperm cell that a machine cannot reliably detect. For an individual sperm cell to be classed as "normal" it needs to be completely normal. Even though some abnormalities do not affect fertility, they still cannot be classed as "normal."

Several of the sperm abnormalities can affect the fertility of the male dog. The sooner any abnormalities are noted the quicker the dog can be managed to avoid possible subfertility.

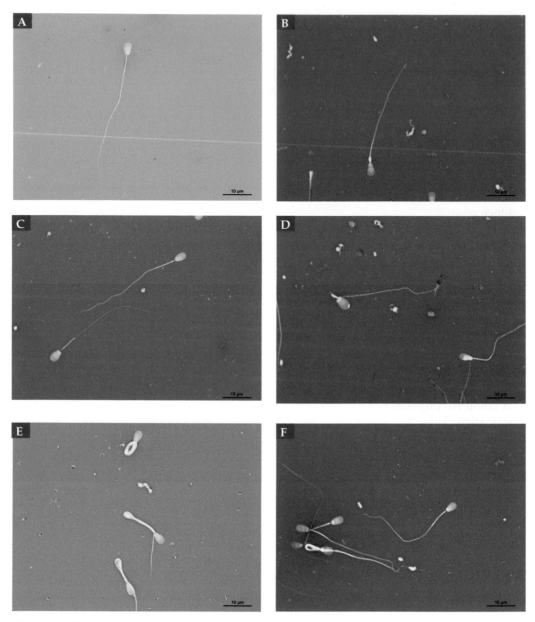

Figure 7.7 Sperm morphology is important in determining the number of normal sperm. A is a normal sperm with a typical head and long tail. B is a sperm with a proximal droplet in the midpiece of the tail. C shows a subtle defect in the sperm head of the uppermost sperm, with a wrinkled acrosome (the very top portion of the head). D includes two defects, one sperm with a misshapen head, the other with an enlarged head that also has a knobbed acrosome at the tip of the head. E includes several with coiled or retroflexed tails. F has multiple abnormal sperm, one has a retroflexed tail, one is dead (pink) and has a 90-degree head formation, and one has a wrinkled acrosome. Photo by JTC.

The percentage of normal sperm cells in an ejaculate usually ranges from 60 to 80%. Dogs are rarely or never over 90% normal, and fully fertile males are commonly in the 50 to 65% range. Any reports that indicate that a male has normal sperm morphology at 85% or above should be approached with caution because the evaluator may have overlooked some sorts of abnormalities.

An additional characteristic of semen that is sometimes reported is viability. This is a measure of how many sperm cells are alive and have an intact cell membrane on their heads. This is very helpful in evaluating sperm cells that have been processed for chilled shipment or have been frozen. Semen samples with low viability can have the breeding dose adjusted to put more live cells into the female during a mating. This strategy compensates for the number of dead sperm cells.

Once all these analyses are completed the evaluator can report on how many normal, motile, sperm cells are present in the sample that was collected. This is done by multiplying the total concentration of the sperm cells by the percent normal and by the percent motile. A breeding dose will depend on the size of the dog but should never be below a total of 100 million normal motile sperm cells. Toy breeds are held to the 100 million threshold, most small dogs to 150 million, medium and large dogs to at least 200 million. It is rare to get more than two to three doses of semen from a single collection on any small to medium dog, so caution is warranted any time a large number of doses are obtained from a single collection. A full report on the analysis should be provided, which should ideally include the details of how the number of doses was obtained. If the report is missing any of the analyses described above, it may be wise to get a second evaluation by another veterinarian.

A complete physical exam of the male dog is part of a thorough breeding soundness examination. This can usually be accomplished most readily after collection of semen to prevent the possibility of a more sensitive male dog being reluctant to ejaculate following a sort of invasive physical manipulation. The physical exam should evaluate all major organ systems and overall general health.

An important part of the examination is palpation of the testes to identify any changes in testicular architecture. Normal healthy testes have a consistency similar to that of a hard-boiled egg, without any wrinkling or firm areas. Any variation in texture should be evaluated further because such changes can indicate testicular degeneration or testicular neoplasia (tumors).

7.6 Processing and Testing Fresh Semen for Shipment

Some dogs are mated by shipping semen to the female rather than by a natural mating. This process uses chilled shipped semen and involves processing the semen after collection. In this situation it is best to have the dog's ejaculate undergo a shipping test about once a year to be aware of any problems that might have arisen. This process involves a full breeding soundness examination, followed by processing the semen for shipping. The ejaculate is evaluated in the usual manner and is then processed with centrifugation after evaluation. This allows for the fluid portion to be siphoned off from the sperm cells. The portion that is natural fluid is then replaced with semen extenders. These are fluids that are specially formulated to protect the live cells for shipping.

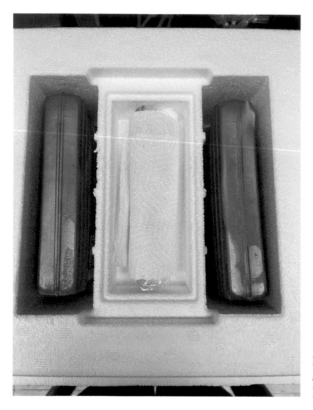

Figure 7.8 Chilled semen is shipped in an insulated container with cold packs. Photo by JTC.

For a complete "shipping test" the semen is packaged just as if it were going to be shipped. The semen is then checked once daily for two days for the various characteristics outlined for routine evaluation of an ejaculate. The shipping test process allows the breeder and veterinarian to select the best extender to be used with an individual dog. The shipping test also provides information on how the semen can be expected to perform when it arrives at the destination.

The test protocol for shipments also identifies individual dogs that might need to have very specific processing requirements for effective semen survival after shipping. Ensuring the accuracy of any processing details required for a specific individual male dog prevents the disappointment of a shipment of sperm that have not survived or is of poor quality. This avoids problems, especially in those situations in which a bitch that has been carefully timed, the owner has diligently ordered semen, has used it appropriately, but then has ended up with few or no viable sperm cells on the receiving end. The shipping test is essential for those breeders that stand a male dog at stud. It is one of the most essential steps the owner of a breeding male can take prior to shipping semen from a dog.

It is unwise to collect semen for artificial insemination as a single collection that is to be used over two or three days. Each day should have a fresh collection. The longer the sperm cells are in an artificial environment, the more they experience cellular damage and the less viable the sperm becomes. The result is lowered pregnancy rates and smaller litter sizes.

7.7 Freezing Semen for Long-Term Storage

Freezing semen is a way to preserve a breeding male's genetics for future generations. While this is theoretically possible, a mating involving frozen semen is neither convenient nor easy! Frozen semen should generally be reserved for use in the somewhat distant future, due to inherent problems in attaining full fertility with frozen semen. In rare circumstances, such as acute illness or injury of the male dog, the use of frozen semen can be necessary even though the dog is still alive and fertile. In general, though, using frozen semen should be avoided if a live, fertile male is available. This is due to difficulties inherent in its use, as well as diminished rates of success when compared to other options for mating.

The most successful age at which to freeze a male dog's semen is between 2 and 5 years old. Performance animals may have not proven themselves by this age, but it is worth getting a few doses in a tank at this age because this is the time window for greatest success. A breeder can then decide later to either keep or destroy the doses. This strategy protects against any unforeseen accident, or against an animal's semen no longer freezing well by the time the animal is proven. This strategy also protects against any other situation that might render the animal unable to mate.

Semen destined to be frozen should have the same full evaluation as fresh live semen. The fluid portions are replaced by fluids designed to protect the sperm during freezing. After these special extenders are added, the semen is then frozen as pellets, in straws, or in vials. Frozen semen should then be thawed and submitted to another full evaluation. Freezing semen puts the sperm through a very tough process. It is taken from the male at body temperature and is then processed with centrifugation and chilled to 4°C in a specialized extender. Following that step it is then exposed to liquid nitrogen vapor or a block of dry ice, and plunged in liquid nitrogen which is −196°C. When the semen is thawed it is brought back up to body temperature in under a minute, prior to insemination. These changes are all potentially lethal to sperm cells.

It is necessary that the sperm cells survive this entire process to assure that the frozen semen will be able to produce a litter. The veterinarian may adjust how many pellets, straws or vials are needed for each breeding based on the outcome of the post-thaw evaluation. A full report with all the associated parameters should be given to the owner at the time of examination. Important considerations include the amount that is being used as a dose, and if the dose has been adjusted for a post thaw evaluation. Frozen semen is a breeding program's future, so it is best to know beforehand if quality is lacking. If frozen semen sounds too good to be true, it likely will be.

Once semen undergoes freezing, it is stored in liquid nitrogen (Figure 7.9). It is then suitable for use indefinitely, on into the future as long as the storage tanks are maintained appropriately. It is recommended that breeders and veterinarians have separate liability insurance on any frozen semen in the event of a catastrophic event at the storage facility or during shipping.

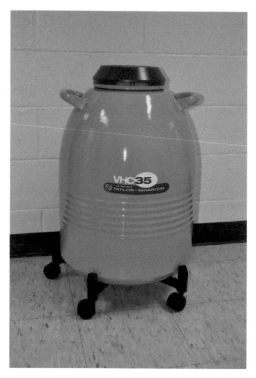

Figure 7.9 Storage tanks for frozen semen contain liquid nitrogen and can store frozen semen indefinitely on into the future. Photo by JTC.

7.8 Key Points

- Sperm cell production takes 62 days from precursor cell to mature sperm.
- Fertility of a male dog depends on events that happened weeks prior to a mating.
- Problems of the prostate gland include hyperplasia and prostatitis and can be managed medically.
- Testicular tumors are relatively common and can affect fertility.
- Breeding soundness examinations can help to pinpoint problems. They evaluate:
  - o libido
  - o ejaculate volume
  - o sperm concentration
  - o sperm motility
  - o sperm viability
  - o sperm morphology.
- Use of semen for artificial insemination with chilled shipped semen requires special procedures for collection and handling.
- Use of frozen semen for artificial insemination requires special procedures for collection and handling.

CHAPTER 8

Management of the Female

The female is the second essential half of the breeding equation. She needs to be healthy to cycle normally, conceive a litter, carry the puppies to term, whelp them successfully, and raise them up to weaning. She is ideally able to do this with minimal intervention and without any complications. Owners can follow a few simple management steps to maximize the chances of a smooth path to a good outcome that ensures their breeding female's success. An important general baseline for success is to keep breeding females current on general wellness examinations and on any health tests that are recommended based on disease prevalence across the region in which the dog resides. Routine examinations and testing should be conducted every year for breeding females.

8.1 Female Growth and Development

As is the case with males, female dogs are born with all their organs formed, even if some of them require further growth and maturation. One major difference between the two sexes is that a female dog is born with the full number of oocytes (egg cells) that will be available for ovulation during her lifetime (Figure 8.1). This contrasts with the situation in males because their sperm production only begins at puberty, at which point cell proliferation begins from earlier primordial germ cells.

Even though dogs produce offspring in litters of multiple puppies, they actually have fewer oocytes when compared to species such as cattle. All the oocytes are in specialized structures called follicles, and all of these are contained within the ovarian tissue. The oocytes reside in quiescent, inactive follicles until the female undergoes puberty. Puberty initiates a process by which sequential cohorts of the inactive follicles undergo maturation and ovulation related to each estrus. More follicles are involved in each of these waves than actually ovulate. This participation of an excess number of follicles may appear to be wasteful but is required because an adequate number of follicles must be involved to maintain the hormonal events necessary to ovulate those few that result in the litter. The follicles not participating in a wave remain inactive and are available for participation in future waves. Sufficient oocytes are present at birth to support estrus and ovulation throughout a bitch's

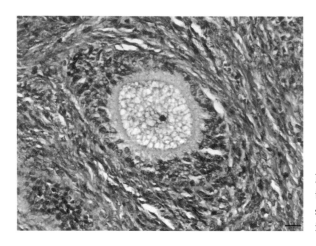

Figure 8.1 Oocytes reside in follicles in the ovary and are surrounded by a rim of small granulosa cells that proliferate early in estrus. Photo by T.E. Cecere.

lifetime, even though the number of follicles is set and does not increase after the female puppy is born.

The age at which puberty (sexual maturity) occurs depends on the final expected size of the mature dog, and as a result it varies considerably from breed to breed. Puberty usually occurs as the dog approaches its expected mature size, at which point she can support a pregnancy and final growth and maturation.

Predicting the specific age at which a bitch will first cycle is difficult. Most females cycle for the first time right around the same age that their own dam first cycled. A certain portion of females that do not cycle before they are 12 to 15 months old have underlying abnormalities, and the use of these females for breeding should be approached cautiously. Females with a late onset of cycles warrant an examination with a reproductive veterinary specialist to determine if she had a silent heat that was missed, or if the animal has any disorder of sexual development. Bitches with either a late onset of puberty or very long intervals between cycles often produce offspring that repeat these same characteristics. As the generations progress, some of the females in these families can have even more extreme delays. This trend must be considered carefully when selecting such animals as breeding stock.

8.2 *Nutrition of the Brood Bitch*

Most of the dietary requirements for bitches are the same as those for males, and the same general principles are valid for both sexes. Commercial canine diets are an appropriate choice in most situations. An entire kennel, from puppies to senior dogs, can be maintained on an "all life stages" diet.

Raw diets – whether frozen, fresh, or dehydrated – are not recommended due to the high risk of contamination with bacteria such as *Salmonella spp.* or *Campylobacter spp.* Both species of bacteria have been implicated in severe systemic infections. In some cases, these infections have resulted in death. These infections are threatening to all dogs but are of most concern for brood bitches. They are especially dangerous during pregnancy and for puppies being weaned.

Some owners prefer to cook for their animals rather than relying on commercial diets. Owners must be sure that any home-cooked diet is well-balanced, and this often requires the aid of a veterinary nutritionist because micro and macro nutrients usually need to be added.

The list of dietary supplements that are known to be safe and possibly helpful for the breeding bitch is very short. Supplements must be used cautiously, with an understanding that they can alter the balanced diet that is already being fed. The following are examples of supplements that may be helpful in some situations.

- Folic acid supplementation is recommended for breeds that are predisposed to midline defects such as cleft palate. The recommended dose is at least 5 mg per animal per day, which is much higher than any product available over the counter. Local compounding pharmacies can make products with sufficient concentration and can make it available to breeders whose dogs need it. Folic acid only needs to be given from the onset of estrus through day 42 to 45 of gestation to have its full effect.
- Glucosamine and fish oil supplements are generally safe to add to a bitch's feeding routine but are only recommended if the diet does not already contain adequate amounts.
- Docosahexaenoic acid (DHA) supplementation can be useful in some situations. DHA is an omega-3 fatty acid that is commonly found in fish. Feeding this during pregnancy can improve the biddability of the puppies. Nutrition experts recommend that bitches be fed a well-balanced diet containing DHA approximately one month prior to their expected estrus, continuing through the ensuing pregnancy and lactation. This assures the maximal influence of DHA on the neuronal development of the puppies. All diets that are labelled for "puppy growth" or "all life stages" have adequate levels of DHA and no additional supplementation is needed.

Although these dietary supplements seem to have beneficial effects, others have generally not been proven to support the female's fertility or improve litter sizes. Prudent owners should carefully read every label and know the ingredients in each supplement that is provided. Nutraceuticals, and this includes most supplements, are not regulated by the Food and Drug Administration (FDA) of the USA, and many of them come with unsubstantiated claims of quality or action. There can be disparities in the actual amounts of ingredients when compared to what is listed on labels.

Aside from the generally vague quality or potential contribution of most supplements, many feed stuffs have been proven to have a detrimental effect on pregnant or actively breeding females. Caution is warranted and these feed stuffs should be avoided. Any other supplements that have been proven to be detrimental should be avoided, even in small amounts. Examples include calcium and products that increase uterine irritability such as raspberry leaf or raspberry extract.

Owners of actively reproducing female dogs should work closely with a veterinarian to be sure that the dog is only being fed products for which the benefit clearly outweighs any risk of negatively affecting the dam or any litter she produces. It is best to closely read product labels for anything being considered for either supplementation or a treatment of a medical condition. Close attention to details assures that an informed decision can be made on the use of any product. Peer-reviewed literature is the best source of guidance on what to feed and what to avoid, and well-informed breeders read this literature first-hand so that they can be confident in what they are feeding.

8.3 Exercise and Fitness

All bitches should be on a routine exercise regimen. This allows for daily socialization and stimulation, and benefits body condition by producing more lean muscle and less fat. Obesity has been documented in several species as altering the metabolic state within the body and producing a chronic inflammatory state, as well as having a direct effect on oocyte maturation. These details have not been specifically studied in dogs, but extrapolation of the findings from other species is reasonable and raises concerns for overweight dogs. Despite a lack of direct evidence, it is best for breeders to keep their dogs at a lean body condition score, 4 or 5 out of 9. This is especially recommended when approaching a mating and throughout the succeeding pregnancy. A healthy body condition needs to be maintained during pregnancy and is especially important prior to mating. It is always healthier and better for the bitch to have to put weight on during pregnancy than for her to need to lose weight. Dietary restriction during pregnancy compromises the growing litter and can be avoided by ensuring the bitch is at an appropriate weight prior to mating.

Exercise assures that the bitch is well-conditioned and fit for parturition. Many performance bitches have easier and shorter whelping periods than bitches that are overweight or less fit. Implementing good cardiovascular exercise well before mating is the best way to avoid dystocia due to an inability to complete whelping due to lack of adequate uterine contractions or exhaustion known as secondary uterine inertia. As little as 20–30 minutes per day of swimming, running, or other form of vigorous exercise produces good and significant results.

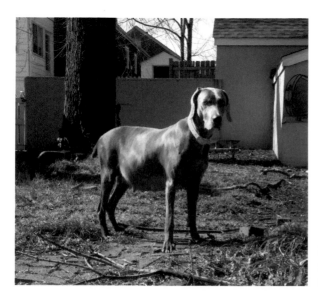

Figure 8.2 In late gestation even the most fit bitch will lose her abdominal tuck. Photo by Meredith Wadsworth.

8.4 *Dynamics of Estrus*

Bitches have four phases in their estrous cycle.

- Proestrus, which is 2–21 days in length.
- Estrus, which is 2–21 days in length and is the phase during which the bitch is mated.
- Diestrus, which lasts slightly over 60 days and is the period of pregnancy or pseudopregnancy.
- Anestrus, the quiet period between cycles, usually ranging from 2 to 10 months.

Proestrus and estrus are commonly referred to as the "heat," and are the two phases that are the most externally obvious because of the physical changes in the vulva as well as the attraction for male attention. Diestrus is relatively quiet from an external perspective despite the important internal changes that are occurring. Anestrus is a period of hormonal and ovarian quiescence. This phase occurs between the end of a diestrus and the beginning of the next proestrus. Anestrus is essential for complete recovery of the reproductive tract for it to be fully prepared for the next cycle.

It is wise for breeders to record each inter-estrous interval (IEI) after a bitch's first estrus. This is the period between one estrus and the subsequent estrus. Most bitches have a consistent IEI, so tracking this gives insight as to when to expect the next heat cycle and helps to confirm that a healthy physiologic process is occurring. Knowing the IEI for an individual dog helps to plan for anticipated matings and can alert breeders to early signs that something is amiss with the bitch's pattern of cycles.

Proestrus is initiated when the brain begins a pulsatile release of hormones that stimulate the ovaries for growth and maturation of follicles. The growth, maturation, and final ovulation of follicles is accomplished by an intricate sequence of gonadotrophin releasing hormone (GnRH), follicle stimulating hormone (FSH) and luteinizing hormone (LH). Follicle stimulating hormone stimulates the growth of follicles. Estrogen is produced from the cells lining each follicle during their early growth.

Table 8.1 The four phases of the estrous cycle depend on ovarian and hormonal changes.

Phase	Ovary activity	Estrogen	Progesterone	Behavior
proestrus	growing follicles	rising	low/absent	attraction by male but female not receptive
estrus	mature follicles, ovulation	falling	rising at ovulation	accepts male
diestrus	corpora lutea	low	rises to day 35, then above 2 ng/ml for about 2 months	pregnant or quiet
end of diestrus	lysis (death) of corpora lutea	low	declines rapidly if pregnant, slowly if open	parturition or pseudopregnancy
anestrus	quiet	low	low	quiet

The bitch enters proestrus under the influence of estrogen. In proestrus and estrus the vulva swells and has a serosanguinous (blood-tinged) discharge. In some females this response to estrogen can result in the overproduction of edema in the vaginal wall, leading to a prolapse of the vaginal mucosa through the vulvar lips (Figure 8.3). Females from some of the shortheaded, thick breeds (Staffordshire Terriers, Pit Bull Terriers, and related breeds) develop this more frequently than other breeds, raising the suspicion that there might be a direct genetic component for the condition, or that it is a consequence of the general conformation of these breeds. Excessive edema with vaginal prolapse creates a management issue as well as a physical barrier to mating, and to whelping because there is an estrogen rise at the end of diestrus. The exclusion of females that have this condition is a wise choice for breeding programs.

A rise in the estrogen levels during proestrus stimulates the release of luteinizing hormone. This transition leads to estrus. Estrus occurs as the luteinizing hormone acts to pre-luteinize and then luteinize the follicular lining cells. It is during this process that the cells lining the follicle begin the production of progesterone and decrease the production of estrogen, which signals the transition to estrus. The spike in levels of luteinizing hormone is the signal for the follicles to ovulate and release oocytes. (Figure 8.4) Following ovulation, luteinizing hormone initiates the formation of corpora lutea (CL) from the ovulated follicles. The corpora lutea produce progesterone for approximately 61 to 75 days, which is the diestral phase of the cycle.

Diestrus has the same hormonal profile regardless of whether the bitch is carrying a pregnancy. This externally quiet phase of the reproductive cycle has very important details. The length of diestrus in dogs is related to hormonal influences that reflect their wolf ancestry. Canine diestrus is a strategy that enables multiple females in the pack to be able to work together to raise puppies. All bitches in a pack tend to cycle synchronously, and then lactate together at the same time. They are therefore all able to help raise the puppies, no matter which of the individual females might be out hunting at any given time. The hormonal profiles of diestrus are the same for pregnant and non-pregnant bitches. In non-pregnant

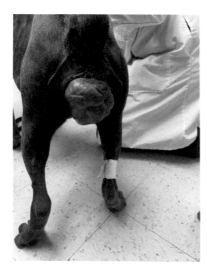

Figure 8.3 Vaginal edema can result in prolapse of the vagina when it is extreme. Photo by JTC.

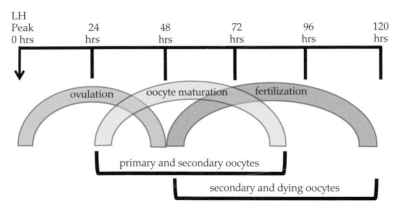

Figure 8.4 The hormonal events and maturation of oocytes occur over a few days. The maximum lifespan for an oocyte after ovulation is 6 days, and most only make it to 4 days. Figure by JTC.

bitches this is called pseudopregnancy, and in many cases is followed by lactation. This relates to the social structure in wolves and is normal. It is no reason for concern on the part of breeders or owners.

A bitch that has been mated and has conceived a litter is then pregnant. At the end of the pregnancy the corpora lutea undergo lysis due to death of the luteal cells. This causes a rapid decline in progesterone levels. The signal for lysis of the corpora lutea is stress signals from the puppies in the uterus. This is one reason litters with fewer puppies are carried for a few more days than those with more puppies. The lack of crowding in the smaller litters provides for less stress, which delays the signal to lyse the corpora lutea. Lysis of the corpora lutea in pregnant bitches occurs between 61 to 63 days after ovulation and culminates in parturition and birth of the puppies.

Bitches that are not pregnant after estrus remain under the influence of progesterone until the luteal cells undergo the lysis that causes cell death and regression. Lysis does occur even in the absence of the signal from stressed fetuses, but in this situation can occur as late as 80 days after ovulation. This is normal, despite it being much longer than a normal pregnancy. The result is that the non-pregnant bitch is under the influence of progesterone for a longer period than is the pregnant bitch.

Progesterone has important influences on the endometrial lining of the uterus. The endometrium proliferates and thickens in both the pregnant and the non-pregnant uterus. In the pregnant uterus this is also accompanied by an invasion of fetal placental cells into the endometrium. In either situation the uterus needs to eliminate excess tissue following diestrus and must then repair the endometrium. Full recovery of the endometrium takes at least two months. The minimum time for an IEI is therefore about 4 months, although the IEI of most bitches is around 6 to 8 months. This allows for 2 months of diestrus and 2 months of repair following the estrus, with time following this for quiescence. Any period shorter than 4 months can result in infertility due to inadequate repair of the endometrium. At the other extreme, the maximum IEI for most dogs is 12–14 months, although this varies from breed to breed. Sight hounds and a few other breeds tend to have longer IEIs when compared to most other breeds of dogs. A veterinary examination is warranted to assure that no underlying abnormalities are present if a bitch is cycling at an interval of less than 4 months, or more than 14 months, between cycles.

The estrous cycle of the bitch can be manipulated by either inducing estrus earlier than it would naturally occur, or by delaying it. This is more generally a theoretical consideration and is only rarely practical. Induction of estrus has been accomplished by several different protocols, none of which can be considered routine due to the timing protocols and the drugs that can be used. One key factor is that estrus should only be induced after a sufficient IEI has occurred (at least 4 months) because hastening the onset of estrus too early has not provided sufficient time for the endometrium to fully recover from the previous diestrus. The chance of conception, and the size of the resultant litter, are both frequently diminished when comparing an induced estrus to a spontaneous one. Conception to an induced estrus is highly dependent on fertile ovulation. Not all protocols are equally successful in achieving this, and individual bitches vary greatly in their response to the different protocols used to manipulate the induction of estrus. Owners that want to mate a bitch during an induced cycle need to accurately follow the appropriate medical protocols and must diligently track hormone levels until ovulation is confirmed. This can take up to a month or more of committed close management.

The methods for delaying estrus vary, and most protocols involve the use of fairly potent drugs. Multiple drugs can accomplish this, and the approval of these varies greatly from country to country. Some of these protocols come at some risk of long-term disruptions of endocrine function in the bitch, and so they must be used cautiously and with close veterinary supervision. It is generally best to skip mating a bitch on an inconvenient cycle rather than delaying the cycle. She can then be mated on her next natural cycle.

8.5 Age at First Mating and Fecundity

The selection of the age at which a bitch should be mated for the first time is controversial, and different people hold different opinions. A bitch's first estrous cycle is a fertile cycle and can produce puppies if she is mated. One detriment to mating bitches on a first, or even second, heat cycle, is that her young age might not have provided sufficient time for complete testing for heritable diseases. Many health tests cannot be finalized until dogs are at least 1 to 2 years old. Full evaluation of temperament and performance are also difficult to assess at a young age. Another drawback is that early mating can diminish an animal's final physiologic growth. More positive reasons for mating at young ages include that this allows for earlier proof that an animal is a good breeding candidate. It also allows her to demonstrate what she can produce. Consideration of all the factors indicates that a good general recommendation is to not mate a bitch until at least the second heat cycle, when health testing has been completed. Deviations from this recommendation are appropriate in some circumstances and can be carefully considered on a case-by-case basis.

Maximum fecundity (prolificacy, or how many puppies are in a litter) occurs in bitches between 2 and 5 years old. After 5 years of age there is a drastic decline in the number of puppies per litter. This occurs even in high-producing lines that are selectively bred for fecundity. This should be considered when planning out a bitch's breeding career, because it may be optimal to mate her prior to her achieving her top titles. Delaying mating may result in smaller litters. The time span for maximum fecundity is an important factor when using frozen semen or when mating to an older or sub-fertile male dog. The combination of an older female and an older male rarely results in a litter of good size or quality.

8.6 Pharmaceuticals

Judicious use of pharmaceuticals is very important for successful dog breeding. The relative risks and benefits of any drug treatment must be considered before its use. Some specific antibiotics have potential negative effects on the bitch and, when used during pregnancy, can have adverse effects on her offspring. The use of antibiotics is appropriate in many cases, but two extremes of their use are to be avoided. The first extreme is the routine use of antibiotics despite a lack of an exact diagnosis of an infectious process. The second and opposite extreme is to avoid all use of antibiotics in any situation.

The use of antibiotics is indeed warranted any time they are indicated for a diagnosed infection. In contrast, placing an animal on an antibiotic without a definitive diagnosis carries with it a risk of inducing antibiotic resistance in resident bacteria. In some geographic regions it has become fairly routine to maintain pregnant bitches on antibiotics even in the absence of a specific diagnosis requiring their use. These regions now have resistant bacteria from the over-use of antibiotics. This resistance then requires the use of other antibiotics to treat common bacterial infections, including antibiotics that have previously been held in reserve to treat more stubborn infections. As improper use of antibiotics increases, more strains of resistant bacteria are created. This eventually leads to an increasingly limited number of antibiotics that will be effective for any infection. Routine use of antibiotics is therefore discouraged. Use should be limited to those cases in which a specific diagnosis indicates their use.

8.7 Common Medical Conditions Affecting Bitches

Every estrous cycle that a bitch undergoes without carrying a litter leads to changes within the endometrium. These microscopic changes mainly consist of cyst formation within the uterine lining. A single cyst is not a major problem, but as cysts increase in number over multiple open (non-mated) cycles they can lead to impaired clearance of the uterus after estrus. This change in the endometrium is called cystic endometrial hyperplasia (CEH). Once the female has cystic changes her fertility will be impaired. This is due to the reduction in the amount of normal endometrial lining that is available for placental attachment.

A further complication of CEH relates to the fact that it develops under the influence of progesterone, which suppresses the immune system. When virulent bacteria gain access to the uterus with a hyperplastic endometrium and increased fluid, the result is often the cystic endometrial hyperplasia-pyometra complex (Figure 8.5). Pyometra means "pus in the uterus" and is a potentially life-threatening condition of the uterus. The combination of hyperplastic changes, fluid in the uterus, and the immuno-suppression related to progesterone makes significant infection and inflammation likely. The age at which this occurs varies, but an intact bitch who has never carried a litter has a high likelihood of developing this condition by an age of 5 to 7 years. Ideally a reproducing bitch will have been successfully mated a few times prior to this age, which diminishes cyst formation within her uterus and

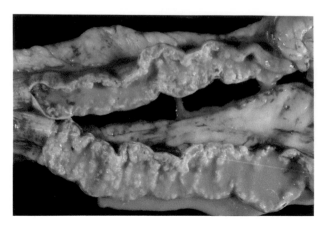

Figure 8.5 Cystic endometrial hyperplasia thickens the inner lining of the uterus and makes it susceptible to infection and pyometra. This opened uterus has the typical thick lining and pus in the lumen. Photo by T.E. Cecere.

therefore limits the chances of developing CEH followed by pyometra. A good recommendation is to mate a bitch while she is young, and then at least once every year or two until she has contributed what is deemed an appropriate genetic mark on her breed. At that point she can have her uterus removed, which also removes the risk of developing pyometra.

Intact bitches that have been retired from breeding should continue to have their cycles tracked and should be watched closely after each heat cycle for at least 90 days. It is important to note any signs of lethargy, purulent vulvar discharge, or increased thirst and urination. An immediate emergency veterinary examination is needed if any of these signs are noted. Although the medical management of cystic endometrial hyperplasia-pyometra complex is possible, it is difficult and should only be undertaken in bitches for which one additional litter is important. Treatment is not without significant risk. The goal is to treat the uterus and mate her on the next cycle. Her uterus should be removed if she fails to conceive. If she does conceive it is still wise to remove the uterus after she weans the puppies.

The only current treatment for CEH is removal of the uterus. If the uterus is not removed, then 80% of bitches that are successfully treated medically will have another cystic endometrial hyperplasia-pyometra event sometime in the next three cycles. Surgical removal of the uterus eliminates any of these problems. A note of caution is that some breeders and owners request that the bitch's ovaries not be removed after her breeding career in light of some evidence that the hormones they produce can decrease the risk of certain tumors and can also increase a dog's confidence and trainability. In this case, if the surgeon is not careful to remove the entire uterus, cystic endometrial hyperplasia-pyometra complex can still occur in the uterine remnant and can be just as life-threatening as it is when the entire uterus is present. The entire situation is complicated. In addition, it is not always recommended to do a hysterectomy on older bitches because the risks can outweigh potential benefits.

Bitches can develop vaginitis, which is an inflammatory condition of the vaginal vault. Vaginitis can result in attraction of males and females. Some affected animals have frequent urination along with some mild cloudy purulent vaginal discharge after urination. No other clinical signs are usually noted. Vaginitis occurs outside of a normal estrous cycle and should not be confused with cystic endometrial hyperplasia-pyometra complex. Vaginitis is common in younger females, usually less than two years old. It is of only minor clinical significance and is more of an annoyance than a serious problem.

Vaginal bacterial flora is present in large numbers in normal animals and are only rarely a cause for any concern. When dysbiosis occurs within the vagina, vaginitis will occur. Dysbiosis can occur peri-pubertally, after dietary changes and stressful events, and if foreign substances have gained access to the vaginal vault. This condition is easily diagnosed via clinical signs, along with inflammatory vaginal cytology (Figure 8.6). Vaginitis must be distinguished from a more serious urinary tract infection (UTI). Vaginitis can give a false impression of a urinary tract infection due to the presence of inflammatory cells. Ruling out a UTI should be done via direct removal of urine from the bladder to avoid confusion with any contributions from vaginal changes.

Vaginitis should never be treated with antibiotics in young animals. Antibiotic treatment only stops clinical signs temporarily but will permanently change the vaginal flora and make the condition worse over the long term. One strategy that can help to resolve "puppy vaginitis" is to add an oral veterinary probiotic to the bitch's daily routine. A second strategy is simply to wait until the onset of her next estrous cycle, because estrus will resolve nearly all cases. If the condition worsens, or does not improve with probiotics after a week, an evaluation by a veterinarian may be warranted. Persistent vaginitis is sometimes related to a foreign body that may have migrated into the vagina and is serving as nidus for infection. Most mature brood bitches do not have problems with vaginitis, so an examination is always recommended if an older female has clinical signs close to her last diestrual phase.

Mammary neoplasia is another condition that affects a large number of intact females. There are two major classes of mammary neoplasia. The first form is benign, or occasionally somewhat locally invasive. This form is cured with removal of the mass and no additional treatments are needed. The second form is much more aggressive and malignant. It can spread to lymph nodes and other organs in the body. Unfortunately, there is no curative treatment for this form and palliative care after diagnosis is the standard of care.

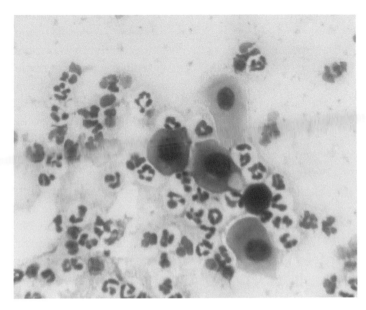

Figure 8.6 Vaginal cytology in cases of vaginitis has neutrophils (small cells with lobed nuclei) along with the expected epithelial cells (larger cells with blue cell bodies and dark round nuclei). Photo by JTC.

The best strategy for managing mammary masses is early detection. Frequently check the bitch's mammary chains. If there is a small mass, have it evaluated by a veterinarian. A fine needle aspirate is not usually rewarding, so an excisional biopsy is a better approach. This is both diagnostic and fully curative for benign mases. Removal also allows for care and management to be tailored for the malignant masses. Mammary masses should be removed and should have histopathology performed to determine if the mass is benign or malignant.

Pregnancy and lactation have not been shown to have a protective effect against mammary neoplasia. Some extrapolation from humans is that women who deliver a baby prior to 20 years old have a significant decrease in mammary neoplasia diagnosis when compared to women whose first pregnancy occurs after 35 years old, or those that have never been pregnant. Brood bitches that have carried at least two to three litters throughout their lifetime only rarely have aggressive mammary neoplasia. This leads to a suggestion, but no proof, that pregnancy and lactation may have a protective effect to some degree. This has not yet been scientifically proven.

8.8 Breeding Soundness Exam

The discussion of a bitch's first mating should begin once she has been deemed appropriate for breeding, has had all her health testing, and has matured into an adult body type. Wise breeders will have a plan for her well before she even hits the ground as a puppy. However, even the best plans need to be revisited and modified as dogs grow, and their traits become more evident. The goal is to benefit the breed and to carefully consider what the bitch could produce with each pairing.

Unlike semen evaluation of the male, it is impossible to evaluate female gametes prior to breeding to see if a bitch is producing normal healthy oocytes in large enough numbers. It is, however, possible to track her cycles and make sure her interestrus interval is within the normal range. It is also possible to document that she has had consistent cycles up to this point in her life. Many breeders will have bitches examined by a veterinarian prior to her first mating. The main important aspects of the exam are a normal wellness check to be sure she is in a good body condition, to be sure she is up to date on core vaccinations, and to perform any other tests that are deemed appropriate for her breed or for the geographic region.

An additional procedure for either maiden or proven females is a digital vaginal examination. This is a vital portion of a physical exam on a brood bitch. The veterinarian palpates the vestibule and vagina to detect any masses, strictures, or structures that may inhibit natural breeding or whelping. Vaginal exam can occur routinely when the bitch is sedated for radiographs and is also reasonably well tolerated by most bitches when they are awake. Vaginal exam gives the breeder and veterinarian a large amount of information before a mating takes place.

Deeper and more thorough investigations are warranted if a brood bitch has:

- missed a conception in the recent past that was deemed her fault
- had dropping fertility such as smaller litter sizes
- some other unusual pathologic condition diagnosed during or after her last litter.

Investigations may include blood tests, ultrasound of her reproductive tract, and vaginal cytology and culture. Any endocrine or inflammatory conditions that need to be addressed can be detected by appropriate blood tests. Any alteration in the normal metabolism of the body will affect cycles and fertility. These should be identified and treated for the benefit of the bitch's health and well-being. Any inheritable conditions should be discussed and her breeding outcome should be based on sound scientific knowledge.

Hypothyroidism is one condition that has been suspected for many years as a cause of reproductive failure in bitches. Very few studies have proven any cause-and-effect relationship. In the most extensive study that has been conducted, bitches who had no thyroidal tissue were able to cycle, conceive, carry to term and whelp their puppies. The only difference between hypothyroid animals and their healthy controls were smaller puppy size at birth, and prolonged whelping. Only those bitches that have confirmed hypothyroidism should be placed on supplementation, and any routine supplementation should be avoided.

Ultrasound examination can reveal possible pathologic changes within the ovaries or uterus such as cystic endometrial hyperplasia or ovarian cysts. Significant changes can be subtle, so the ultrasonographer should be specifically skilled and experienced in looking at the canine reproductive tract. Breeders need to recognize that not all pathologic changes are large enough to be seen via ultrasound. A negative result does not always mean that there are no abnormalities present.

Vaginal cytology and culture of the cranial vagina or uterus are other procedures that could potentially be conducted. Cytology reveals the presence of inflammation and needs to be interpreted along with results from the bacterial culture. Bacterial cultures are difficult to interpret because normal bacterial flora is present in both the vagina and the uterus. The result is that nearly all cultures lead to positive growth, because nearly all animals have normal bacterial flora. The bacterial species present in the normal flora are not a cause of concern except very rarely, so interpretation of cultures should be done cautiously. In rare situations dysbiosis has occurred in which the balance of bacterial species is upset. In other cases, there can be contamination of the vagina and uterus with a virulent strain of bacteria. Both situations can lead to bacterial overgrowth and clinical disease.

Bacterial culture requires the use of a guarded swab to avoid contamination with the bacteria that are normally present in the vestibule of the vulva (Figure 8.7). An alternative to a guarded swab is endoscopic equipment that can accomplish low-volume lavage of the uterus. Both techniques lower the risk of aberrant results. Accurate results are important to avoid any improper use of antibiotics. Antibiotics are only needed in very few cases, and understanding the dynamics of the normal bacterial population helps breeders to reduce inappropriate uses of antibiotics. Some owners of male stud dogs require proof of a negative culture for bitches that are presented for mating. In those situations, the bitch's owner should collaborate with the veterinarian to decide if this practice is truly necessary or if it is even warranted at all. As an alternative to this, many veterinary reproductive specialists provide evidence to concerned breeders that there is no clinical indication for routine vaginal culture on bitches. They decline to do the culture procedure because it is unnecessary and rarely leads to any accurate diagnosis or management.

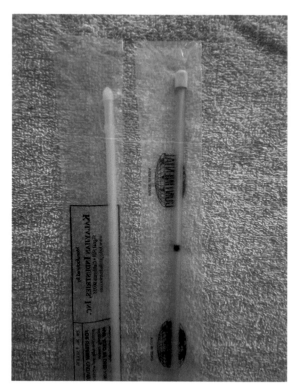

Figure 8.7 Guarded swabs have caps over the shaft of the swab that prevent contamination from tissues that are external to the anterior vagina. Most of these are about 60 cm long. Photo by JTC.

8.9 *Frequency of Pregnancy*

Mating a bitch over multiple successive cycles can reduce fecundity. This is especially true when the cycles occur in rapid succession. Cycles that occur every 4 or 5 months are more frequent than normal, resulting in drastic changes both in the endometrium and in the general metabolic state. The relatively short number of years that a bitch has maximal fertility makes it tempting for breeders to maximize the litters that can be obtained from her to reach their goals for their breeding program. This requires careful consideration of the frequency of her cycles along with the relative amount of genetic material she should contribute to the breed.

A bitch can metabolically handle two matings on successive cycles if these occur every 4 to 8 months. She cannot recover as well on a third pregnancy at this frequency. Breeding a bitch this often may result in a loss of fertility, or a complication with the pregnancy or lactation.

The consequences of back-to-back mating are less drastic for a bitch that is cycling every 9 to 12 months. This interval provides a longer time for her systemic health to recover when compared to shorter intervals. Planning ahead and having clear goals for an individual bitch and her genetic contribution to the breed can allow for a few back-to-back pregnancies, ideally followed by an unmated cycle. This pattern can be repeated multiple times and will still allow her to recover metabolically. If a bitch cycles rapidly a discussion of delaying her heat cycles can also accomplish a longer interestrus interval. This is complicated to do and not commonly done specifically for breeding purposes.

The brood bitch is very important to a breeding program. She provides half of the fertility and genetic contribution, but unlike the male she must actually carry the pregnancy, whelp on her own, and raise her young. Her multiple roles in successful reproduction make her management more complex than that of the breeding male, so her management is best prepared well in advance of an anticipated mating. Keep careful records on health testing, vaccination status, and cycle intervals. Bitches that are in good body condition and have daily socialization and stimulation raise the best puppies. These simple steps will assure for kennels to be successful in managing female lines.

8.10 Key Points

- Bitches are born with their full complement of oocytes.
- The estrous cycle is a complicated cascade of changing hormonal signals.
- Pregnant and non-pregnant bitches all undergo similar hormonal changes, and pseudo-pregnancy is normal for unmated bitches.
- The non-pregnant uterus is at risk of cystic endometrial hyperplasia and possible pyometra.
- A bitch's breeding career should be carefully planned as to age of onset, frequency of mating, and eventual retirement.

CHAPTER 9

Management of Mating

The general goal of dog breeding is for the bitch and sire to produce litters easily and with an appropriate number of puppies in the resulting litter. Success can be achieved naturally, but also through a variety of artificial or assisted techniques. Every step away from a fully natural situation tends to diminish the final outcome, and this must be considered carefully when planning the protocols for mating and breed maintenance. Success depends on careful planning and good decision making (Figure 9.1).

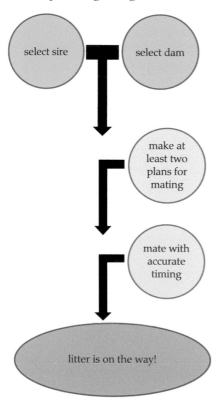

Figure 9.1 Successful production of a litter depends on several decisions along the way. Figure by JTC.

Maximizing success in situations where artificial means are used requires accurate timing and a general knowledge of the techniques that are available. A team-based approach with the veterinarian and the dog owners is an essential starting point. Advances are continually being made that improve the outcomes for assisted reproduction in dogs. While assistance is possible, the reasons for it have profound consequences. Assistance due to scheduling or spatial complications has very different consequences when compared to that for situations that use it to circumvent behavioral or fertility challenges in the lines of dogs being bred. The consequences that assisted reproduction can have for the long-range maintenance of a dog breed need to be carefully considered before such techniques gain wide acceptance and use.

Mating two dogs is obviously essential to produce a litter of puppies. The specific way in which the mating occurs can vary and all of them succeed best when a detailed plan is used for accurate timing of the mating. Even the most common protocols for mating dogs demand a good plan, and advance planning works to a breeder's advantage. Experienced breeders never claim that mating dogs is convenient! Often a mating will have to happen over a holiday or during some other pivotal life event. This sort of inevitable snag needs to be kept in mind, and plans can take this into account to minimize complications. Owners of male breeding dogs need to be very clear and specific about when that dog is available for mating, and when he is unavailable. Bitch owners also need to communicate clearly when their female is expected to be in season, and need to be prepared to adjust accordingly when expectations change.

One important baseline is to be sure that all breeding animals are up to date on vaccinations and general health care, as well as on brucellosis testing. These basic components need to be in place well before the mating is scheduled to take place. It is never good to need a vaccination at the last minute, or to find out that a bitch has an active infection when she goes into estrus, or that a male has a problem when he is required for mating services.

Owners of male dogs need to communicate to clients the scheduling of any other bitches to be mated around the same time as the client's animal. Healthy males may be able to cover two females in rapid succession within a day or two, but this should be only done with a good degree of caution as it is not the best practice. Daily sperm output is the number of sperm cells the testes can produce per day. Males with daily ejaculations have diminished daily sperm output, regardless of whether these ejaculations are through mating or through semen collection. Daily sperm output is higher in those dogs that are allowed to rest at least one to two days between ejaculations. Male dogs can only produce about 20 million sperm cells per kilogram of body weight. A mating dose is between 100 and 200 million normal motile sperm cells, and daily sperm output depends on the mature size of the animal. There are only so many cells that a male can produce per day and this number is heavily influenced by the frequency with which he is mated or has semen collected.

Breeders need to be sure they have multiple plans in place in case something goes wrong, or the first plan does not work out. Secondary plans might include skipping a cycle or referring the bitch to another male. These alternatives need to be decided as possibilities prior to any mating. Veterinarians specializing in reproduction are greatly frustrated when their help is requested to salvage a poorly prepared plan, with the consequence that a breeder needs to scramble and hastily assemble an alternative plan during the optimal time window for a specific mating.

Once a specific pair of dogs is identified, breeders need to decide on how the mating will take place. Depending on the method of mating, this will require arranging any travel accommodations, shipping companies, or veterinary hospitals that will be used for timing and insemination. Communication among all three parties, the two dog owners and the veterinarian, will ease the entire process.

Planning ahead includes considering time of year, ease of raising puppies, and any performance events where a breeding dog may be expected to compete. Bitches in season are not allowed to compete in most performance events. Looking ahead to the schedule of those events will take careful observation. For example, a conflict can arise in situations where it is desirable to breed a hunting female on her next cycle, but her national field trial will occur right about the time she is due in season. In this situation the breeder can:

- plan ahead, intending to skip the trial and mate the bitch
- delay the bitch's heat cycle with the help of a reproductive specialist, compete her, and then mate her on the subsequent cycle
- discuss inducing a heat cycle in enough time to allow for the bitch to be mated, whelp, and raise a litter in advance of the big trial.

The first two options are routinely viable, very dependable and are well tolerated. The last, induction of a heat cycle, is more difficult, more expensive, and can have side effects. Induction may not even result in a fertile cycle despite the use of expensive drugs and time. Due to induction's unpredictability, it is better to plan in advance and either accomplish the mating and skip the trial or delay mating until the next heat cycle.

Further complications can arise when male dogs are in a place where neither natural cover nor semen collection and shipment is possible. Communicating this to owners of bitches is important. Frozen semen is always an alternative but comes with significant expense and lowered success rates. Similar complications can arise with sudden illness or injury to the male dog. Communication is key, and owners of breeding bitches should always have an alternative plan in place just in case it is needed.

9.1 Timing the Mating

The single most important factor in successfully mating a pair of dogs is the timing of the insemination, regardless of the specific method by which this occurs (Figure 9.2). Most of the infertility cases that are presented at reproduction referral facilities are due to improper timing. Timing is everything when it comes to mating dogs, and breeders should go to great lengths to assure that sperm cells and oocytes are in the same place at just the right time. Much of this depends on the individual cycle of the female and on the male's breeding schedule.

Choosing a female that has normal cyclicity is a huge benefit to timing. Females that have irregular cycles often end up with reduced or non-existent fertility. The same is true of females that have not had at least four months between from the last heat cycle and the intended breeding cycle. Fertility is also likely to be low in females at the other extreme, with irregular cycles that have over twelve to fourteen months between them.

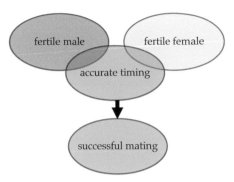

Figure 9.2 Successful conception of a litter requires not only a fertile male and a fertile female, but also requires accurate timing of the mating. Figure by DPS.

The frequency with which a male is used for mating is also an important factor in timing. Dogs are different than other species, and some common practices used in other species often fail with dogs. Splitting an ejaculate for use in multiple females is a common practice in horses, and rarely works with dogs. Mating an individual male dog to two or more females on the same day likewise needs to be avoided.

9.1.1 Oocyte Maturation

Several factors that are unique to dogs influence the timing of fertile mating (Figure 9.3). Each of these occurs over a stretch of time rather than at a specific easily identified point. These include:

- ovulation
- maturation of oocytes
- survival of sperm in the female's reproductive tract.

Ovulation and oocyte maturation in the bitch are directly related to the rate at which the progesterone levels rise in the bitch. The follicular lining of dogs undergoes luteinization

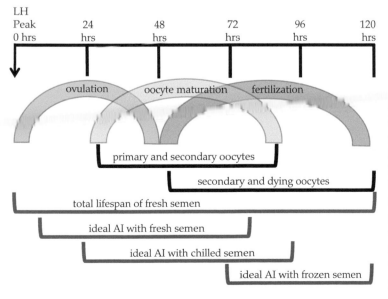

Figure 9.3 Ovulation is followed by maturation of oocytes, and this process influences the ideal time of insemination by different protocols. Conception can occur outside of these time windows, but maximum success occurs when mating is within these periods. Figure by JTC.

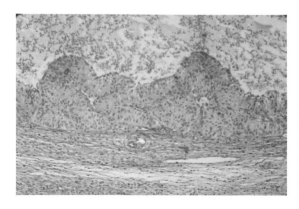

Figure 9.4 The lining of a canine follicle becomes thicker and lined by plump cells prior to ovulation, which indicates a change from estrogen production to progesterone production as the cells luteinize. Photo by K. McEntee.

before ovulation, a process called "preluteinization" because of the contrast with the pattern in other species where luteinization occurs only after ovulation (Figure 9.4). As the follicles luteinize prior to ovulation, progesterone production rises. The follicles within a cohort do not ovulate simultaneously, but instead ovulate over a short period of time that can last up to a day or two. Breeders and veterinarians can track a cycle's progression by measuring progesterone levels, which helps to optimize the timing of mating or insemination.

Progesterone levels are easy to track. The key to accurate timing of insemination depends on the rate at which the follicles and oocytes mature, and these events are related to a rapid upward trend in progesterone that occurs over 48 to 72 hours. This is referred to as the "progesterone curve." Documenting this hormonal trend is the key to accurate timing of mating. A common misperception is that ovulation reliably occurs when progesterone concentration reaches some specific level. This is incorrect, because it is the upward trend that is more important than the absolute level of progesterone. Relying on a specific absolute level can lead to a poorly timed mating. Ovulation in response to the peak can occur over a wide range of absolute progesterone levels. Progesterone levels (over time) need to be combined with other information to know the tight window of maximal fertility. Three things need to be kept in mind.

- Bitches ovulate their oocytes over several hours or days.
- Progesterone levels, and especially the upward trend in values, assist in tracking the cycle and determining the time of ovulation.
- Ovulation and oocyte maturation is related directly to the steepness of the progesterone curve and not to an absolute level of progesterone.

Bitches are unique among mammals because they ovulate primary oocytes. These are not capable of immediate fertilization, in contrast to the situation with other mammals that ovulate secondary oocytes. Two meiotic cell divisions occur between the time of ovulation and the time of conception, and both are required to produce the secondary oocytes that are prepared for fertilization. These divisions can take anywhere from 24 to 72 hours after ovulation, and when they occur is related to how rapidly the progesterone levels are rising. The process of oocyte maturation gives breeders a distinct advantage but can also be a challenge. Canine oocytes live in the reproductive tract for approximately 4 to 6 days after ovulation, and during this window they can be fertilized if they have achieved the status of secondary oocytes.

9.1.2 Different Methods for Timing

Multiple strategies can be used for timing a mating. Each of these has strengths and drawbacks. They all rely on the underlying hormonal changes that occur during estrus (Figure 9.5). These include:

- progesterone levels (currently the most available method)
- levels of luteinizing hormone
- cytology
- vaginoscopy.

The ovaries of a bitch in proestrus contain follicles that are growing and that produce estrogen. Estrogen causes edema (tissue swelling) of the vulva and vagina. It also allows for diapedesis (leakage) of red blood cells through the walls of the uterus. This blood-tinged fluid is expelled through the vagina and out through the vulva. Proestrus is the early part of the cycle and the point of highest estrogen production. After proestrus the bitch goes into estrus, at which point the lining of the follicles progress to a stage of pre-luteinization that occurs before ovulation. The luteal cells in the follicular lining begin to switch from estrogen production to progesterone production. Progesterone levels can be used as a tracking mechanism to fairly accurately pinpoint ovulation because they rapidly spike, right at the time of ovulation. Luteinizing hormone is the specific signal for the follicles to begin the change from estrogen production to progesterone production. Luteinizing hormone is produced within the pituitary gland at the base of the brain. Levels of luteinizing hormone rise in response to large amounts of estrogen circulating in the body. Luteinizing hormone acts to luteinize the follicles as well as causing them to ovulate the oocytes that are contained

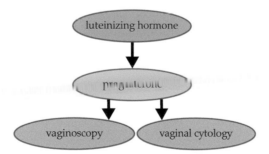

Figure 9.5 A mating can be timed by noting changes in several different events that cascade from one to the next. These begin with luteinizing hormone, go through an increase in progesterone, and finally result in changes in the vaginal lining. It would be most accurate to time a mating by measuring luteinizing hormone levels as this is the factor that is closest to the original onset of the cascade. However, due to limitations in procedures for measuring luteinizing hormone it is not practical to do so. As a result, measuring progesterone is the most practical compromise for ease of measurement, while retaining a good level of accuracy. Figure by DPS.

within each growing follicle. Ovulation usually occurs 24 to 28 hours after the spike in luteinizing hormone.

Luteinizing hormone is unfortunately a fragile molecule that breaks down quickly in the body. The consequence of this is that measuring luteinizing hormone levels, despite its usefulness, is not practical in most situations because timing scenarios based on luteinizing hormone levels require daily measurements. No commercial test is currently available to quantify the amount of luteinizing hormone, so understanding this detail of hormonal control is of more theoretical than practical use. There is a semi-quantitative procedure for detecting luteinizing hormone, but this provides only a result of "present or absent" and not a specific level. The fragility of luteinizing hormone is the reason that progesterone, which is a much more stable molecule, is the better method for tracking most cycles.

Progesterone begins to be produced as the follicles pre-luteinize in response to luteinizing hormone. Levels of progesterone in the blood can be monitored periodically to track the trend of these levels, remembering that the goal is to document the rapid spike in levels. The rate at which oocyte maturation occurs is directly related to the rate at which progesterone rises. Progesterone is released in a pulsatile manner and follows diurnal rhythms, so it is best to sample bitches in the morning and at a consistent time each day. Measurements should start on day five or day seven of the cycle, with day one defined as the first day that blood is observed in the vulvar discharge. Continue sampling every other day or every third day until the progesterone spike (causing ovulation) is confirmed. This protocol allows for reliable comparisons of the levels, as well as providing sufficient time to notify the owner of the male if semen is to be shipped.

Typically, the surge in luteinizing hormone will begin to occur at around a level of 2 ng/ml of progesterone and ovulation will occur anywhere between levels of 3 and 10 ng/ml of progesterone. At least one blood sample should be analyzed for progesterone 24 to 48 hours after a suspected ovulation to complete the hormonal curve accurately as it related to the timing of the mating. Quantitative measurement of progesterone is essential for matings that will require shipment of fresh semen, or any use of frozen semen. Accurate detection of ovulation allows for accurate determination of pregnancy milestones and ultimately a due date for whelping, which can be very helpful at the other end of the pregnancy.

Progesterone levels are measured by several different testing methods, each with its own relative accuracy. Many different machines and methods are currently available for these measurements. It is important to know which specific method is being used to track a bitch's cycle, and the relative accuracy of that method. The method based on radioimmunoassay is the most accurate and was previously the standard to which other methods were compared. Radioimmunoassay has inherent risks to laboratory personnel because it is based on radioactive components. As a result, it is currently only used in research settings.

A second method is currently more broadly available and relies on chemiluminescence as a quantitative measurement of progesterone. This method has been extensively compared with radioimmunoassay and has now achieved equal accuracy. Chemiluminescence is currently considered as an accurate and reliable method of progesterone measurement. Despite the inherent reliability of this technique, not all machines that do this test function equally as accurately. Each machine has its own margin of error. Owners and veterinarians need to work closely together to determine the amount of error that is acceptable during a mating.

The top-end machines that are used for chemiluminescence progesterone measurement have very low variation over multiple samples as well as minimal variation in results when a single sample is tested multiple times on the same machine. These machines are very accurate, with reliable results that correlate well with the radioimmunoassay method. One of these top machines is the IMMULITE™ machine from Siemens. A few factors make this machine an impractical choice in some settings. It has a high initial cost and has complex control methods that are required for its use. In addition, this machine requires a fairly long run time for each sample: about 45 minutes from the time serum is placed on the machine until the result is available. Most veterinarians in general practice will not have access to this machine, and consequently many other machines have been introduced to meet the need of breeders. Any machine that is available should be independently validated against a radioimmunoassay or a chemiluminescence machine because both methods are validated as accurate for use in canine species. Additionally, radioimmunoassay and chemiluminescence have appropriate standards of variance both within a single sample and between several samples. Validation of a machine ensures that the machine has repeatable and consistent results not only with itself, but also with other machines of the same type.

Within a single estrous cycle, it is unwise to switch between either the method or the specific machine used for progesterone measurement. Sticking to one method and one machine avoids the poor correlation that multiple methods or machines can have with one another. One method and one machine should be used throughout the entire mating event, even if the final insemination takes place at a different location. Reference laboratories that evaluate send-out samples generally use the same machines as most of the large universities. This ensures that the results have consistency over large numbers of samples.

Progesterone levels can be drastically altered by additives to the tubes in which the blood is collected. It is essential to only use plain glass tubes with no additives. Problems can easily arise when the wrong tubes are used for collecting the blood samples. Successful matings can be missed due to inaccurate progesterone numbers, so every effort must be made to assure consistency regarding time of sampling, collection tubes that are used, the method that is used, and the machine providing the results.

Vaginal cytology was widely promoted as a fairly reliable method for timing the mating of dogs in the days prior to the availability of documenting progesterone levels. Cytology is no longer considered accurate enough for this purpose because it is less accurate than progesterone levels at clearly defining ovulation. Cytology's usefulness is limited to determining the presence of estrogenic influence and any inflammatory process. Vaginal cytology is accomplished by sampling cells from the vagina with a cotton tipped applicator, rolling them onto a glass slide, staining them, and then examining them under a microscope to characterize the proportions of different populations of cells in the sample. Several illustrated guides for this method are available and can help in the interpretation of the results. These guides illustrate the presence and proportions of the typical cell types that are present during each of the stages of an estrous cycle.

Vaginal cytology relies on the effects of hormones on the vaginal wall. Under the influence of estrogen, the vaginal epithelium (surface lining) increases the number of cellular layers to prepare for mating. The increased number of layers provides an enhanced barrier to trauma during mating. The change in the layers can be tracked by changes in the proportion of the various sorts of cells that are present (Figure 9.6).

Parabasal cells come from the deepest cell layers, and these are usually only two to four layers thick. Over these are the superficial epithelial cells, and the number of layers of these increases during the cycle to produce 20 to 40 layers. The rate at which this thickening happens, as well as other changes to background debris and other cells, is very dependent on both the individual bitch and the individual cycle. Cytology is usually only tracked clinically by veterinary reproductive specialists if the cycle is prolonged or otherwise aberrant. Unfortunately, there is no tight correlation between vaginal cytology and the time of ovulation.

Vaginal cytology is very effective in revealing any inflammation in the vagina and is therefore useful despite its limitations in accurately reflecting the time of ovulation. Inflammation is evident when the presence of non-epithelial cells, such as white blood cells, occur in high numbers. This finding has no correlation to ovulation and should not be used alone in attempting to time the mating of a female (Figure 9.7).

Vaginal cytology can be useful to help determine an accurate whelping date. After ovulation and oocyte maturation the epithelium in the vaginal vault undergoes a reverse in the proportions of cell populations seen during estrus. This is due to high progesterone levels and low estrogen levels that are typical during pregnancy. As a result of these shifts in hormones, the female goes from having a majority of superficial epithelial cells to a drastic shift towards parabasal cells. This shift is called the diestral shift, and noting the day of this shift can assist in determining a whelping date. Experienced veterinarians should be able to assist with the reading of the cytology slides.

Vaginal cytology is especially helpful in predicting a whelping date in those bitches that will require a caesarian section but are also useful in situations where incomplete or no progesterone timing was performed. For this strategy to work successfully, the cytology sampling needs to start when the bitch is in estrus. Only then can the technique pinpoint the date at which the proportions of the various cells shift. Once the shift has occurred, cytology is no longer of any use because the proportions then remain relatively constant.

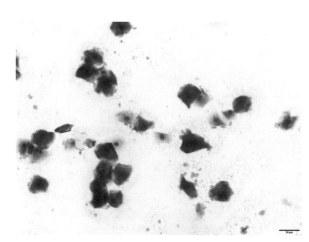

Figure 9.6 Vaginal cytology is not highly accurate but does have the advantage of being quick and accessible in most locations. Under the influence of estrogen, the darker blue keratinized cells predominate over the parabasal cells that are pale and have obvious nuclei. Photo by JTC.

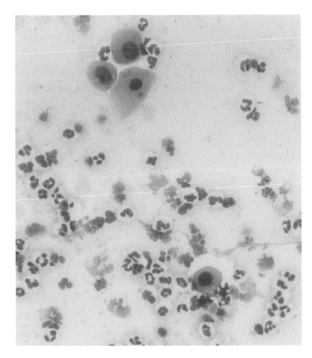

Figure 9.7 Cases of vaginitis have numerous neutrophils in addition to epithelial cells. Photo by JTC.

Vaginoscopy is another technique that can be used to track the changes in estrogen influence over time. The vaginal canal responds to the changes in estrogen levels within the body. High levels of estrogen increase the edema (swelling) of the vaginal walls and produces a "pillow" appearance of the folds within the vaginal canal (Figure 9.8). As estrogen drops and progesterone rises the vault changes its appearance to flattened and crenulated folds, much like that of a runway at an airport (Figure 9.8). This can be a valuable tool for tracking bitches who are having unusual progesterone trends or are not progressing normally through an estrus. Specialized equipment is involved with this procedure. The equipment ranges from a full endoscopic camera to specialized proctoscopes or altered otoscopes so that their length is adequate to reach the cranial vagina. This allows visualization of the folds, which is essential to the success of the technique.

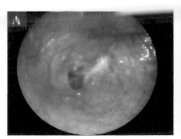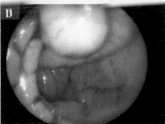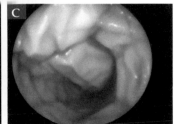

Figure 9.8 The vaginal wall changes over the estrous cycle of the dog. Image A shows the wall during anestrus, with a flat epithelium. Image B shows the wall in proestrus. Image C shows the thickening and edema of the wall during estrus. Photo by JTC.

Accurate timing of mating is essential when trying to minimize the number of insemi-nations that are required, and to maximize conception rates and litter sizes. Understanding the physiologic process that occurs in the bitch during estrus is the key to understanding the basis for the different methods by which the cycle can be followed, to use them to their maximal benefit. The most fertile days of a cycle, and the ideal time to mate, vary some-what depending on the type of semen being used (live fresh, chilled, frozen) and on the relative fertility of the male. Breeders and veterinarians that are well-versed with track-ing technologies and semen handling generally are more successful at producing fertile matings.

9.2 Methods of Mating

The most successful approach to dog reproduction is for a live fertile male to be mated naturally to a live fertile female. Every step away from this natural situation diminishes the final success rate for conception and litter size. The alternative to natural mating is artificial insemination, whether by semen freshly collected, shipped chilled semen, or frozen semen.

Pairs of breeding dogs can mate by many different procedures. Each one has its own subtle details that need to be considered every time a mating is planned. The details influ-ence the amount of semen that is placed within the female for each mating, and this has a large influence on the conception rate. It takes more than one sperm cell to actually produce a puppy. The collective effort of many sperm cells on a single oocyte is required to assure the penetrance of the one successful sperm cell that conceives the puppy. Because of this aspect of group activity, it is generally true that increasing the numbers of live, motile sperm improves the outcome.

When young fertile females and young fertile males are mated naturally, peak fertility occurs somewhere between days 10 and 14 of the cycle most of the time. Even in this most favorable situation, natural mating succeeds only about 80% of the time. When natural mating occurs during an unmonitored estrous cycle there is no information as to which specific day the bitch ovulated, or on how quickly the oocytes matured. When these details are not monitored it can affect the chance of conception and litter size, and lack of this information also makes it more difficult to calculate pregnancy milestones such as expected date of whelping. The life span of sperm in the female reproductive tract indicates that multiple matings separated by a day yield the maximum chance of viable sperm and mature oocytes both being present at the same time and in the same place, which is the essential ingredient for successful conception.

Some bitches that are presented for reproductive diagnostics due to infertility have been mated several times without success. They are then labeled as infertile or sterile. Many of those bitches never had documentation of progesterone levels as an aid to timing the mating. Some of these bitches may have ovulated in the first week of estrus. Others wait to ovulate well past day 20 of their cycle. While extreme, neither of these situations is abnormal. Other variations include bitches that have split heat cycles. Such animals do not have a fertility problem, and any reproductive failure is related to timing of mating and not inherent infertility. Animals with split heat cycles require close monitoring to suc-cessfully conceive a litter. Individual bitches are usually consistent through every cycle.

Another important detail to consider is that bitches that are housed together in kennels tend to cycle together. The individual bitches in that situation are prone to either being delayed somewhat or pulled into an estrus early due to "the dormitory effect" that is influenced by their kennel mates.

The behavior of the dogs being mated also influences the choice of mating method used. Some very dominant alpha bitches will never stand for a natural mating. Some submissive bitches will stand no matter where they are in their cycle. Standing behavior generally occurs when levels of estrogen are falling, and progesterone levels are rising. Unfortunately, the behavior of a bitch is not always an accurate indication of ovulation. Male behavior in response to the female can also be inaccurate as an indication of ovulation. Timing of mating based on progesterone levels and the progesterone surge, in contrast, is always accurate. The most accurate approach to the timing of mating, and the best chances for successful conception, is to time the mating based on progesterone levels that have been monitored over the entire length of the estrus. This is especially important in bitches that have proven difficult to successfully mate.

A few techniques surrounding the mating of dogs are commonly used, but some of them have little positive influence on outcomes. Regardless of the mating method used, the female does not need to be restrained from sitting or urinating after breeding or insemination. Sperm that are motile swim through the cervix in as little as 30 seconds from insemination and are therefore where they need to be well before the bitch has time to sit or urinate. After vaginal insemination, the elevation of the hindquarters of any bitch does not need to occur for any longer than one minute after the insemination. One practice that can be helpful is to routinely use that short time to digitally stimulate the vaginal canal before letting her down to a standing posture.

9.2.1 Natural Live Cover

The best pregnancy rates and the largest litter sizes are achieved when natural matings are performed every other day for the entire length of the fertile days of an estrous cycle. Natural live cover is the most successful method for mating dogs, but obviously requires that the dogs be in the same physical location for a few days. It is always best to have the female travel to the male, or to meet in a neutral location to avoid consequences of any territorial behavior. Semen from a fertile male will last 5 to 7 days in the female's reproductive tract and will be ready to fertilize the oocytes as they mature

If the dogs are in close proximity, mating every other day until the female is no longer standing is best. This may be unrealistic because many dogs are not that close in proximity. Typically, two matings, with 1 day off in between, should occur between 1 day before ovulation and 3 days after ovulation. Progesterone timing should continue throughout this period, ideally with the same technology and machine used for each measurement. A day off in between matings allows for additional sperm cells to be deposited within the female at the second or third mating, ensuring that sufficient viable sperm are present for the oocytes as they mature.

Live cover should occur in a natural environment free of any distractions. Dogs with good libido will have no problems figuring things out if they are size-matched and allowed to run freely for a few minutes prior to mating. At least two people should be present, one to hold the female if she will not stand still and another to assist the male if he needs some help. If the male is smaller than the female a ramp or step can be helpful in aligning the penis with the vulva. Lubrication that is free of any spermicidal ingredients should also be available if needed. It is important to note that KY jelly or any lubricant with chlorhexidine will kill sperm cells, so these must be avoided.

Once mounting and intromission have occurred, the male will begin fast rhythmic thrusting. The male will then dismount from one side and turn around in the opposite direction, forming a copulatory lock or "tie" (Figure 9.9). Once tied the pair cannot be separated manually without risking injury to both dogs. The male may need assistance in getting his hind leg over the female's hindquarters during the turn. This lock allows for the occlusion of venous blood flow and maintains his erection. The female assists in maintaining the lock. The sperm-rich fraction of the ejaculate has usually been expelled before the time of this turn. The remainder of the time during the lock the ejaculate consists of jets of prostatic fluid, which is not sperm-rich but does cause increased pressure in the female's vagina and forces the previously ejaculated sperm-rich fraction of semen through the cervix.

Most natural ties last anywhere from 15 to 45 minutes. The female determines the duration of the tie. If a tie lasts longer than an hour, the dogs need to be immediately examined by a veterinarian to avoid potential serious damage to the reproductive organs. Breeding accidents have happened during natural cover, but rarely occur when mating is attended because the people in attendance can intervene if needed. It is important for those attending to not be impatient or rough.

One way to assist with natural matings is to use mild anxiolytics in those females or males that are too timid or too dominant to participate in the process. Finding a veterinary reproductive specialist that is willing to do an assisted natural mating is extremely helpful to any breeder. This also allows for evaluation of natural breeding behavior as well as maximizing numbers of sperm obtained from a male. Natural mating provides for maximum numbers of sperm cells. Even experienced male dogs that are accustomed to being artificially collected do not produce the same high number of sperm cells in a collection as they would deposit during a natural mating.

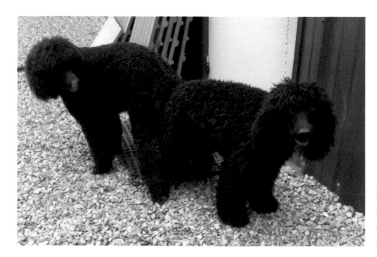

Figure 9.9 The "tie" is a normal part of the sequence of canine mating. Photo by Susan Tapp.

9.2.2 Artificial Insemination

Artificial insemination is increasingly common as a strategy for mating dogs. The three usual methods for inseminating the bitch include:

- vaginal artificial insemination (VAI)
- trans-cervical insemination (TCI)
- surgical artificial insemination (SAI).

Each of these methods is appropriate for some situations and not for others. The variables include the individual dogs being mated, the techniques used to prepare or handle the semen, and the availability of trained personnel to accomplish the technique.

Vaginal artificial insemination requires the use of a long pipette that is gently manipulated up through the vaginal vault to the level of the cervix. This delivers semen where it is deposited in natural live cover. When done correctly it places the semen far enough cranially to be effective and does so without any loss of valuable semen. If done improperly, rough inseminations can lacerate or even perforate the vagina and cause infections. The bitch's cervix sits under her lumbar spine, well beyond the pelvis. A note of caution for anyone doing inseminations at home is to remember that this is not a risk-free procedure. The risk of negative outcomes is real, and best avoided by having the procedure done by someone specifically trained and experienced with it. The vaginal artificial insemination technique is only used with fresh or shipped chilled semen and is not successful with semen that has been frozen.

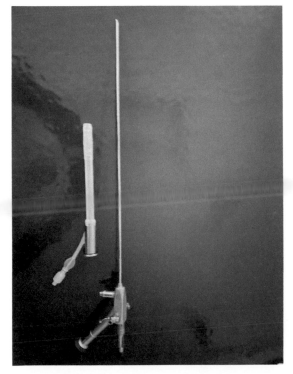

Figure 9.10 The pipette used for trans-cervical artificial is long and thin, and accurate placement is aided by insufflation of air through a larger hollow shunt. Photo by JTC.

Trans-cervical insemination requires specialized equipment that deposits the semen directly into the uterus by going through the cervix with a cervical catheter (Figure 9.10). Trans-cervical insemination gets the semen just a bit farther into the reproductive tract but requires a veterinarian to perform the procedure. One trans-cervical insemination method uses a rigid endoscope and camera for visualization of the cervix and the catheterization. Lacerations and perforation of the vagina may occur if the female moves suddenly or sits on the scope. Breeders need to be aware of the expertise of the person who is performing these types of inseminations due to the possibility of complications. Experienced specialists include many that almost exclusively use trans-cervical insemination with the rigid scope. They have had great success with no complications, so the element of safety is more related to experience and ability than it is to the choice of equipment.

Surgical artificial insemination requires surgical entry into the abdomen under general anesthesia. Semen is then injected directly into the uterine lumen. This is abdominal surgery, and it has potential complications that are inherent to any abdominal procedure. Potential complications need to be taken very seriously. Entering the abdomen of any animal is a major surgery and no animal should have more than three elective abdominal procedures during its life. Each surgery induces inflammation, scar tissue and possible formation of adhesions. All these postsurgical sequelae can result in life-threatening conditions.

The relative advantages of trans-cervical insemination and surgical artificial insemination are debated heavily. The cost and expertise to perform these two procedures are very different, and each has advantages and disadvantages. If all things are equal (such as semen quality, fertility of the female and timing of insemination) then pregnancy rates and litter sizes are equivalent for the two techniques. Trans-cervical insemination has the advantage of not requiring sedation or anesthesia in most cases. Trans-cervical insemination takes less than twenty minutes, and the bitch then walks out and goes back to her normal daily routine. Surgical artificial insemination requires general anesthesia that carries its own possible complications, requires a sterile environment, and takes about an hour or more from start to finish. The female undergoing this procedure also has exercise restrictions post operatively.

Both trans-cervical and surgical artificial insemination deposit semen in the uterus. Some facilities limit the use of surgical artificial insemination for those cases where it is desired to actually visualize the uterus, to take uterine biopsy samples, or when some malformation of the reproductive tract is suspected, and it is necessary to document the abnormality. If a bitch can only conceive with surgical artificial insemination, then it is important to ask if this is something that should be propagated within the blood line. Surgical artificial insemination is an invasive procedure, and some veterinarians refuse to do it unless there is some specific medical reason that requires it.

When comparing surgical artificial insemination and trans-cervical artificial insemination, it is generally better to find a veterinarian that performs the trans-cervical procedure. When that is not an option, encouraging a veterinarian to go to a continuing education course to learn how to perform a trans-cervical artificial insemination is a good strategy. Trans-cervical insemination is an additional skill that will bring business and expertise to the practice. The main advantage of trans-cervical artificial insemination is that it avoids an elective abdominal procedure that is unnecessary.

9.2.2.1 Side-by-Side

A side-by-side insemination is when the male and female are in the same facility but are not allowed to mate naturally. Reasons for this can include:

- an injury or size disparity in one or both of the dogs that may cause concern for a natural mating
- an alpha bitch that will not stand for a natural mating
- a female that has a very prominent urethral papilla or abnormal vaginal conformation that makes it difficult for the male to gain intromission.

The side-by-side technique consists of collecting an ejaculate from the male with the female present. The collected semen is then used for insemination. The semen should be placed in the female on the same timing schedule as that used for natural mating. This is typically one mating per day for two matings, with 1 day off in between. These should be accomplished between 1 day before ovulation and 3 days after ovulation. Measurement of progesterone levels should continue throughout this period to optimally time the mating. The levels should be ideally measured with the same method and machine for all samples.

The degree of processing for semen used for a side-by-side mating varies and depends on the protocol favored by the personnel doing the collection and insemination. This varies from minimal processing all the way to use of semen extenders. In most situations the collected semen is deposited in the female either by vaginal artificial insemination or by transcervical insemination. Any time that semen is collected it is wise to evaluate it so that the quality of the male's semen can be determined and documented. This can give valuable insights into any changes that occur over time.

9.2.2.2 Shipped Chilled Semen

The use of shipped chilled semen is becoming increasingly popular as a strategy for breeding management. As breeders become more globally dispersed, and individual dogs are separated by large geographical areas, exchange of genetic material is easiest to manage through artificial means. Dog breeders find that shipped chilled semen is a good way to accomplish this. With this strategy, the male's semen is collected, evaluated, processed, and mixed with extenders that protect and sustain it. It is then shipped overnight at refrigeration temperature. Not every delivery company can deliver every day of the week or on holidays, and this is a potential constraint on the timing of collection and shipment. Shipped chilled semen has allowed genetic diversity to be spread large distances with very little financial outlay due to the ability to avoid the shipping or transporting of live dogs. Timing the use of shipped chilled inseminations varies greatly and final schedules are based on:

- the number of inseminations requested
- when the insemination needs to occur
- the quality of the semen being shipped.

It has become commonplace for semen collected by the owner of the male dog to be shipped. This strategy should be used with at least some caution. Many of the possible problems that can arise with this technique can escape detection if a collection is not evaluated at the time of collection or again at the time of insemination. Any males that are producing semen to be shipped and chilled should have test shipments and evaluations performed periodically to assure the quality of the product at its destination. Accurate and current evaluations make it easier to adjust for any upcoming matings and can alert breeders to any potential problems well before there are missed conceptions.

Shipped chilled semen should be inseminated anywhere between 1 day before ovulation and day 3 after ovulation. Progesterone timing should continue throughout this period, ideally with consistent technology. Typically, the semen needs to be available the day of ovulation or the day after. This first insemination can be reinforced with a second shipment that occurs on day 2 or 3 following ovulation. If only one insemination is going to occur, insemination one or two days after ovulation is adequate. Semen can remain viable in the female for 5 to 7 days, even if it has been shipped, so insemination should occur the day the semen is received. If additional inseminations are wanted, a second shipment should be obtained. Sperm cells never survive equally well on the bench top as they do in the reproductive tract, so quality of shipped chilled semen drastically declines 24 hours after collection. This remains true despite additives to the extenders, addition of new extender, or other interventions meant to enhance sperm survivability. The best place for semen is in the bitch. This semen can be deposited by the same procedures used for fresh semen, depending on owner preference.

9.2.2.3 Frozen Semen

Using frozen semen for dog reproduction has several significant challenges and success rates have been variable. Resorting to frozen semen should be reserved for situations when a male dog's genetic influences will be wanted in the future after the dog is gone, no longer fertile, or has had an acute injury and is no longer available for natural service. Any mating based on frozen semen is a risk and there are a few important details that an owner needs to consider before using frozen semen in a breeding program.

- A significant commitment needs to be in place for very accurate timing of ovulation. Frozen semen must be inseminated when the oocytes are ready to be fertilized because the thawing process shortens the life span of the semen to about 12 hours. This means that the owner must commit to monitoring progesterone or luteinizing hormone and must follow through completely and accurately.
- Even though a male was producing puppies at the time his semen was frozen, this does not guarantee that his frozen semen will be of sufficiently good quality to remain fertile after thawing. The highest success rates come from frozen semen from a male that has already produced puppies with frozen semen. This is especially true when all the collections were done within a reasonable time. If one collection was performed when a male was 2 years old, another at 5 and the last one at 8, it is unlikely that all will be similar regarding post-thaw quality.

Breeders that rely on frozen semen, including both the owner of the male dog and the bitch, should be diligent to require semen evaluations. Any evaluation should have all the components included in routine semen evaluation. Evaluations should also have comments about post-thaw quality. Frozen semen should be reserved, if possible, for females that have had at least one litter in their recent past and that are still young and fertile, usually between 2 to 4 years of age. Using unproven frozen semen in a maiden female has a high risk of failure. When an unproven female fails to conceive following the use of frozen semen, it is impossible to know if the fault lies with her, with the semen, or with the timing of the insemination. When a failure occurs, the breeders lose the expected litter, one or more doses of semen, and the estrous cycle of the bitch.

For adequate fertility, frozen semen must be placed directly into the uterus 3–4 days after ovulation by either trans-cervical insemination or surgical artificial insemination. Inseminating on both of those days does not increase the chances of a pregnancy, so one or the other of the days is sufficient. Insemination at the correct time requires careful timing and may warrant a multimodal approach. Some facilities routinely use trans-cervical insemination when using frozen semen. It can be routine to use two doses of frozen semen per insemination until the semen from that male is proven to have conceived a litter. The greater the number of normal, motile sperm cells available, the higher the chance at success. Once the frozen semen from a male has produced puppies it is possible to use one dose per breeding. This ensures that enough normal, motile sperm are available to perform the task. Breeders should work closely with a veterinarian to help make decisions to move forward with this type of insemination. When purchasing frozen semen, it is important that specific questions are asked.

- Has frozen semen previously produced litters?
- How many different collections are available?
- When was the frozen semen proven?
- How was the semen previously used?
- What was the evaluation at the time it was frozen?
- What was the evaluation after it was thawed?

9.3 Dual-Sire Mating

Dual-sire or multi-sire mating is the practice of having more than one male mate with a female during a single estrous cycle. This has become an increasingly popular strategy over the past few years, largely because accurate pedigrees are now possible through DNA testing of sire, dam, and puppies. One mistaken impression is that the two sires used to mate a bitch will each end up producing 50% of the litter, or in the worst case a deviation that does not exceed a 75% to 25% split. This theoretical expectation is simply not true in most cases. Only about 30% of litters following dual-sire matings result in puppies being produced from both sires. Even in that 30% of litters where both sires contributed, most litters will have only a single puppy from one of the sires, with the rest of the puppies from the other sire.

The reasons for this uneven contribution of sires occurring are complicated. One important factor is that lower quality semen (even if from a highly desired male) will always be outcompeted by higher quality semen, even if the lower quality semen is placed in the female first. One erroneous recommendation sometimes made is the use of dual-sire situation for valuable semen that is in low quantities. The idea behind this is that the semen from the other male will assist the semen from the low-quantity male. In this situation it is important to remember that the low-quantity semen may well be able to conceive a litter on its own, but if it has to compete with semen from another male, it may well end up not producing any puppies. In that situation, the valuable semen has been wasted.

Another consideration is that semen from multiple different sires introduces an increasing amount of "non-self" cells that are placed in the bitch. This increases the chance that the bitch will generate an immune or inflammatory reaction to the introduced sperm cells. Any negative reaction within the uterus or uterine tube will negatively impact the success of the mating. The current recommendation for a dual sire breeding is to choose males of similar fertility. Even in that optimal situation, it is still highly unlikely that the litter will end up being sired by two different males, much less one having an even split of puppies produced from two sires.

Regardless of success rates, the parentage of the puppies from any dual or multiple mating needs to be proven with DNA testing of the puppies. This is essential before the puppies can be accurately registered.

9.4 Key Points

- Mating needs to be timed carefully to assure maximum fertility.
- Timing of mating is important:
  o bitches ovulate in response to a surge in luteinizing hormone
  o bitches ovulate over a period of a few days
  o oocytes mature over a period of a few days
  o semen, especially fresh semen, is viable over several days in the female reproductive tract.
- The male or female reproductive tract is the safest place for semen.
- Progesterone monitoring is the most accurate of the practical ways to pinpoint ovulation.
- Mating procedures include several options:
  o natural mating
  o side-by-side artificial insemination
  o shipped chilled semen
  o frozen semen.
- Each step away from the natural situation diminishes overall results.
- Using multiple sires in a mating is rarely successful.

CHAPTER 10

Management of Pregnancy

Canine pregnancy is relatively short and is the critically important period that takes a litter of puppies from conception through to birth. During pregnancy, several factors constantly undergo changes. Most of the dynamic action is occurring deep within the bitch's body, concealed from the caregivers. It can be a very stressful time for breeders and owners because they must prepare for a litter, tighten biosecurity in the kennel or home, and adjust quickly to the ever-changing needs of the pregnant bitch. Breeders need to be prepared for what is to come, while supporting the changes in the body of the pregnant bitch so that she can make a smooth transition from pregnancy into whelping and then raising the litter. Major problems during pregnancy can be warded off with swift identification of any emerging problems, as well as veterinary examination at least twice during the pregnancy.

Pregnancy is generally divided into thirds called trimesters, and each of the trimesters comes with its own host of needs and risks. Puppies develop quickly during pregnancy and undergo several important developmental milestones in each of the trimesters (Table 10.1).

During the first trimester the initial conception of a puppy occurs as the sperm and oocyte fuse and unite their genetic material to produce the puppy's genotype. This first single cell then multiplies into many, which then differentiate and assemble themselves

Table 10.1 Each trimester of pregnancy has different stages of puppy development and unique risks.

Trimester	Events	Risks
first	embryogenesis organ formation	teratogens high levels of radiation drugs a few nutrients (vitamin A)
second	organ growth slow body growth	drugs trauma some infections
third	final more rapid growth	inadequate nutrition of dam

into the various organs of the body. The developing puppy is most sensitive to a wide variety of potentially damaging influences during the early stages of organ development, and this period is the one most prone to serious mishaps.

The second trimester is relatively quiet when compared to the other two. The organs that developed in the first trimester continue to grow, although somewhat slowly. The risk during this period from the influence of infectious agents and consequences of any toxins is lower. Managing the first two trimesters of pregnancy are fairly easy because there is minimal risk of disease transfer to the puppies. Despite the relative safety of these periods, precautions should still be in place to safeguard the bitch and her health.

The last trimester is the final three weeks of gestation. During this period, the puppies undergo their period of final growth, which occurs more rapidly than over the first two trimesters. This is also the period of maximum metabolic demands, and the period of most concern over any infectious disease agents.

Biosecurity of the kennel and the individual pregnant bitch are important throughout the entire process of mating and pregnancy and is essential in the last trimester. Throughout all trimesters the pregnancy is sustained by the hormone progesterone. One characteristic of progesterone is that it suppresses the bitch's immune system. The immunosuppression occurs right along with all of the dynamic metabolic changes in the pregnant bitch's body, leading to a level of increased risk for both dam and puppies. Breeders can help protect both the dam and the litter by providing a safe and clean environment in which gestation can occur.

Every pregnant bitch should be up to date with her vaccines. This ensures that the dam can defend her own body from the most common infectious threats that she is likely to encounter. In addition, her own protection is eventually transferred to the puppies during late gestation and early after birth. A further precaution is that pregnant bitches should be kept away from any dogs of unknown vaccination status. This can be especially challenging in a relatively open kennel that has dogs going to and coming back from shows or other events. The same is true of kennels that temporarily board dogs, or that add new dogs. In kennels that are relatively open, the more transient dogs should all be placed under some sort of quarantine that precludes their potential to interact with pregnant bitches. All new arrivals should be quarantined for at least four weeks to minimize any opportunity for disease transfer.

Heightened biosecurity is especially important in the third trimester. Any exposure to canine herpes virus is especially risky during these weeks, and this virus is widely prevalent in most populations of dogs (Figure 10.1). Up to 90% of dogs in some parts of the world have tested positive for this virus. The herpes virus is especially devastating following its introduction to a kennel that has previously not been infected. The canine herpes virus is readily transmissible from dog to dog through saliva, nasal secretions, semen, and the fluids and tissues that result from an abortion. Bitches that have not been exposed to herpes virus prior to mating are susceptible to infection. The outcomes of infection are especially bad in the third trimester, when infection with the virus can result in death of portions of the placenta and fetal tissues. This can result in outright abortion of the litter, or the birth of stillborn or weak puppies. Simple biosecurity measures are the best way to alleviate transfer of this disease to pregnant bitches.

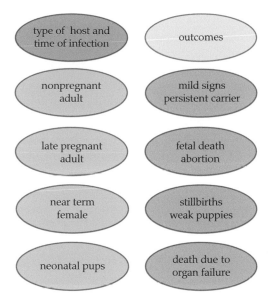

Figure 10.1 The consequences of an infection with canine herpes virus depend on the age, immune status, and reproductive state of the host. Figure by DPS.

Although herpes virus is especially hazardous during the third trimester, any disease that causes clinical illness in a pregnant bitch can negatively affect the pregnancy and the litter. Pregnant bitches should not be travelling to shows or competitions and should be kept away from any animals that are new to the kennel or that are travelling. The best recommendation is to shut down the kennel for the last three weeks of gestation and for the first three weeks after the birth of the puppies. Isolation avoids the risk of communicable diseases and becomes even more important after the birth of the puppies. While no canine herpes virus vaccine is available in the USA, a vaccine is used in Europe and can minimize the risk of the disease to adults and to their puppies.

10.1 Nutrition and Supplements

A few details of diet, nutrition, and supplements are specific to pregnancy. Several nutrients are especially important:

* docosahexaenoic acid (DHA)
* folic acid
* calcium (too much or too little are both problems)
* vitamin A (too much is a very big problem).

Appropriate commercial diets are well balanced for needed nutrients in appropriate amounts. They are also closely monitored for quality control, and therefore are very unlikely to contain high amounts of any toxic ingredient. "Balance" is the key concept in nutrition for pregnant bitches. Some owners are tempted to provide an excess of many nutrients that may well be essential when present in their appropriate amounts. Excess of many of these can unbalance the diet, and this can be especially dangerous to developing puppies and pregnant bitches. Pregnancy is an especially poor time for thinking that if a little of something is good, then more is better.

Docosahexaenoic acid (DHA) is necessary for optimal neuronal development of the puppies as they develop during the pregnancy. Feeding a diet rich in DHA results in biddable, responsive puppies. Bitches should be on a diet that has adequate DHA prior to breeding. If the diet does not have DHA supplementation, a pregnant bitch should be switched immediately to a diet labelled for all life stages, or to a puppy formulation.

Folic acid supplementation may be necessary for those breeds that are pre-disposed to midline defects, or for any bitch that has a history of producing midline defects in previous litters. Folic acid supplementation should start at mating and should continue through day 42 to 45 of gestation, under the guidance of a veterinarian. The required amount of folic acid is not easily provided by over-the-counter formulations, so the source and formulation are important details.

Calcium supplementation is not necessary if the bitch is on a commercial diet. Calcium supplements that are over generous actually disengage the body's ability to mobilize its own calcium stores. This can be life-threatening immediately after whelping because the bitch needs to mobilize calcium quickly to produce milk. The hormonal system that mobilizes calcium from the bones and other tissue stores needs to be intact and functioning well as the bitch transitions from pregnancy to lactation. Generous calcium supplementation during late pregnancy can actually defeat this purpose rather than helping it because such supplementation diminishes the bitch's ability to mobilize her calcium stores.

Bitches with a decreased appetite, or that vomit any calcium supplement, are at risk for hypocalcemia (low blood calcium), especially in the last two weeks of gestation when the puppies have their most rapid growth and require calcium to mineralize their bones. It is best to rely on the commercial diet to provide the needed nutrition instead of relying on additional supplementation. A veterinarian can assist in deciding if a bitch needs any calcium supplement during pregnancy in addition to what is present in formulated diets.

Diets that are too rich in vitamin A have been shown to cause midline defects (Figure 10.2). Chicken livers and some other foods are especially rich in vitamin A. While it is very important to not over-supplement any nutrient in the bitch's commercial diet, this is especially true for vitamin A. It is especially tempting to feed chicken livers to finicky pregnant bitches to stimulate appetite and food consumption, but it is important to find other foods that will encourage her to eat. It is also important to ensure that what she does eat is well balanced.

10.2 Exercise and Fitness

Exercise is very important to the pregnant bitch. Exercise keeps her body in lean shape and allows for daily socialization. Many body changes occur in the bitch as she progresses through her pregnancy, and some of these may be surprising to inexperienced breeders. There is a loss of abdominal muscle tone. The abdominal tuck typical of a dog in ideal body condition disappears because her abdomen enlarges with the pregnant uterus (Figure 10.3). This is further developed by a loss of muscle tone and relaxation of ligaments and tendons.

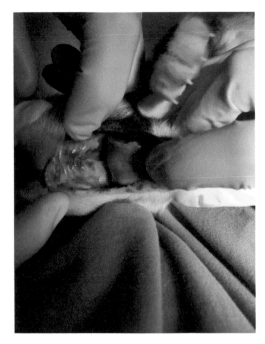

Figure 10.2 Supplementing vitamin A can result in cleft palates among the puppies of the litter. Photo by JTC.

A pregnant bitch should have her normal exercise routine for the first month after she is mated all the way up until she is checked for pregnancy. Strenuous work at this point does not have a negative impact on fertility rates or litter size. Swimming is great exercise throughout pregnancy and there is no risk to causing a uterine infection if a mated or pregnant bitch is allowed to swim. Barriers are present in the vagina and uterus that prevent any contamination that could arise from ascending fluid or bacteria.

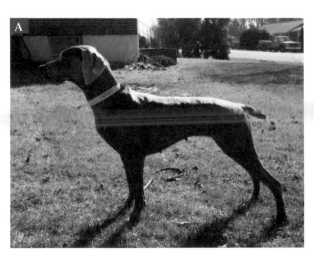
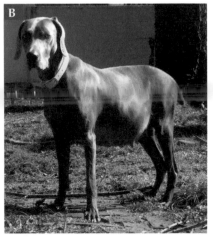

Figure 10.3 A bitch in late gestation loses the abdominal tuck she had when not pregnant. This is the same bitch in a fit, non-pregnant status (A) and in late gestation (B). Photos by Meredith Wadsworth.

Later in pregnancy, especially in the last two to three weeks, the bitch should be allowed to dictate her own tolerance level of exercise. An example would be a bitch that usually walks two miles daily but then begins to slow down after only one mile. This is normal and appropriate. Some performance dogs self-run 10 to 15 miles (15 to 20 km) at an average rate of 5 to 10 miles an hour up (7 to 12 km/hr) all the way up to the day they whelp. These are bitches that are extreme athletes and that are accustomed to this level of strenuous exercise. They tolerate it well and in addition they enjoy it. Bitches in good athletic condition whelp easier and faster than their lazier counterparts. The important issue is to not allow a pregnant bitch to be too lazy, while at the same time ensuring that in later pregnancy she is allowed to determine when she is tired and is not pushed beyond her limit.

10.3 *Pregnancy Diagnosis and Monitoring*

Pregnancy diagnosis has evolved over the years and has become an important part of successful dog breeding. The unique nature of the hormonal curves of the bitch makes it easily possible for a breeder to be fooled into thinking that a bitch is pregnant even though she is not. To avoid managing non-pregnant bitches as if they were pregnant, most bitches should have some form of a pregnancy check around mid-pregnancy. This is on or near to day 28 after ovulation. A few different procedures can determine if a mating produced a pregnancy and can ideally alert a breeder to the approximate number and viability of the puppies.

One method for pregnancy diagnosis is ultrasound, which has become highly valued due to its accuracy (Figure 10.4). An ultrasound examination can be done by any veterinarian who has access to an ultrasound machine. This provides a wealth of information and is safe as well as relatively fast. Ultrasound provides an image that reveals structures deep into the body. It distinguishes densities of fluid from the various sorts of solid tissues such as fat, muscle, and bone. Ultrasound examination can reveal the fluids and developing puppies within the uterus of the pregnant bitch.

Ultrasound examination is generally performed between days 21 to 30 after ovulation. Experienced and capable ultrasonographers can see fetuses as early as 14 to 16 days. Ultrasound waves are safe and do not cause any harm to the developing puppies. In addition to a "yes or no" diagnosis as to pregnancy, it is possible to determine if the fetuses are viable due to the ability to observe heart flutters. Ultrasound examination can also identify any problems with the pregnancy or with an individual fetus. It is not unusual for a pregnant bitch to resorb a single fetus, but if several are being resorbed then it is wise to pursue further diagnostics as well as instituting procedures for managing a high-risk pregnancy. An estimate of litter size may be made, although ultrasound is only 30% accurate at predicting the number of puppies. This is due to the nature of ultrasound, the high mobility of the uterine horns, and the potential for continued fetal loss after the time of diagnosis.

Ultrasound examination also allows veterinarians to be able to take specific measurements of fetal structures as an aid to determining gestational age. In experienced hands these measurements can be very accurate and help to determine a due date for whelping. This is especially true in cases in which the bitch has not had levels of progesterone monitored to provide an estimated day of ovulation. Some publications have documented

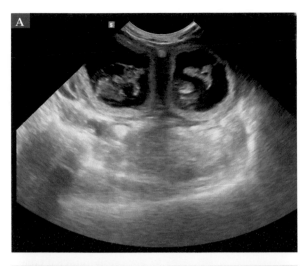

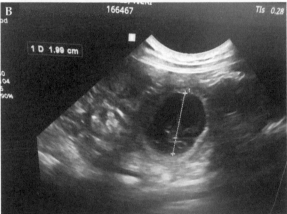

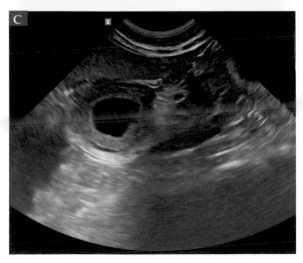

Figure 10.4 Ultrasound probe that images that allow a fetus to be visualized inside its fluid-filled sac within the uterus. In image A the fetus is still viable and within its fluid, image B shows how measurements of the fetal/placental unit can be used for aging the pregnancy, and image C reveals a fetus that is being resorbed, with disruption of the fetus that should be in a fluid filled sac. Photo by JTC.

successful determination of fetal sex prior to whelping, although the accuracy decreases exponentially with the size of the litter.

Blood levels of the hormone relaxin can also be used as a pregnancy test. Relaxin is produced by the placenta of the fetus and can be measured by a commercially available test on a blood sample from the bitch. This test only gives a "yes or no" answer as to pregnancy. Unfortunately, it can have results that are either false positive (a nonpregnant bitch with a "pregnant" result) or false negative (a pregnant bitch with a "nonpregnant" result). The test has limitations due to a threshold of a minimum detectable level of relaxin. Small litters or singletons can produce a negative result because they are not producing enough relaxin to reach the threshold level of detection. Fetal demise will also affect the result. The placenta remains present and functional in some cases of fetal death. This can result in a positive test despite the lack of a viable pregnancy. Despite these drawbacks, testing for relaxin levels has been widely used with success, although breeders need to be aware of its limitations and the information that will be lacking when it is used alone without other diagnostic approaches.

Abdominal palpation is another approach for pregnancy diagnosis. An experienced person can feel an enlarged uterus, as well as the fetuses resembling a "string of pearls", around 28 days after ovulation. The "pearls" are the developing puppies, each within its fluid-filled placental sac. Once the bitch is past 35 days of gestation the fetuses enlarge, and the fluids increase to the point that each placental/fetal unit butts up against its neighbors. At this point they feel as if they have merged, and the palpator can no longer detect individual puppies. At this stage, the pregnant uterus can be easily confused with other abdominal organs. There is no reliable way to determine the viability of the developing puppies by palpation. Counting puppies using this approach is very difficult and often inaccurate.

Radiographs can also be used for pregnancy diagnosis. This modality requires the use of radiation, so while it is very useful for counting puppies prior to whelping, it is not ideal for early pregnancy diagnosis. Fetal skeletal mineralization does not begin until after day 42 of gestation. Prior to this, any radiograph will reveal only a mass effect that will be unable to differentiate between fluid or puppies within the uterus. The bones of the puppies start to mineralize around day 42 of gestation, but at that stage of development the bones are still only faint on radiographs, and therefore counting the puppies remains difficult. Radiography in pregnancy is best reserved for use one week prior to a due date. At that point, a radiograph is useful for counting fetuses in preparation for whelping. Studies have shown that radiographs at this point in pregnancy are a safe practice and can be performed without detrimental effects to dam or fetus.

10.4 Parasite Control

Nearly all bitches harbor both round worms and hook worms. The larvae of these parasites often remain in a quiet and inactive state within the body tissues of the bitch. During pregnancy there is a reactivation of these parasitic larvae. They migrate through the mammary glands of the bitch where they are then available in milk. They also migrate directly through the placentas of the fetuses and into the fetuses themselves.

The parasitic infection of the puppies through this mechanism can be drastically reduced by deworming the bitch during pregnancy as well as after whelping (Figure 10.5). The goal is to reduce shedding and transmission of the parasites to the puppies. This reduces the parasitic load that the puppies will carry after they are born and minimizes any damage caused by these parasites during the development of the puppies in the uterus.

Currently there is a lack of specific evidence that bitches on monthly heartworm prevention have adequate prevention against the migration of the parasites other than heartworms. In the absence of such evidence, it is best that all bitches be dewormed during pregnancy. Two methods have been found to be effective.

- Daily deworming from day 41 of gestation to day 14 post-partum prevents reactivation and migration of the parasitic larvae. This protocol is not very practical and is rarely chosen by breeders because of the amount of the drug that is required and the requirement for daily administration.
- A three-day deworming protocol using fenbendazole at day 41, 42, and 43 after ovulation. This drastically reduces the larval migration and the infection of the puppies. Combining this with a deworming protocol starting at day 12 post-partum for both puppies and their dam, will ensure that a litter has a very low parasitic load. This protocol also prevents any zoonotic transfer of larval parasites to humans.

10.5 Pharmaceuticals

The use of any prescribed medications during pregnancy should be approached with caution. Pharmaceuticals have been closely studied in many species, and can be classed as:

- known to be safe
- should be used with caution during pregnancy
- unsafe and should not be used during pregnancy.

Drugs are allocated a grade of A through D, where A designates those drugs known to be safe, and D designates those known to be detrimental. Grades A and B are safe to use

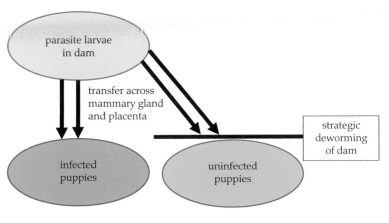

Figure 10.5 Strategic deworming of pregnant bitches greatly reduces parasite loads in puppies. Figure by DPS.

in most situations, while grades C and D need to be used with extreme caution. The grades are noted in most formularies that are available. Veterinarians can use the grades to guide decisions as to which drug is safe or best to use.

Clinical situations may arise during a pregnancy that require specific treatments. If treatment is warranted be sure that the veterinarian consults with reproductive safety data or any comments on toxicology prior to prescribing a pharmaceutical medication. The benefit must always outweigh the risks, and use of any drug should be limited to situations where drugs are absolutely necessary instead of as a routine practice.

At around the time of pregnancy diagnosis, 28 days or so after ovulation, many bitches will become finicky eaters or might stop eating all together. There is currently no explanation for why this happens, but most of the time it is easy to remedy. The antacid famotidine has been used for many years and is safe for use during pregnancy. Famotidine is considered a category B drug for pregnancy and lactation. This drug helps reduce the acid within the stomach and is well tolerated by pregnant bitches. Using this drug usually resolves the reluctance to eat within the first 24 hours of administration. A veterinarian can help to arrive at the correct dosage and should also be consulted if the bitch does not respond to treatment. In this event, an examination of the bitch is prudent. Appetite stimulants and antiemetics (anti-vomiting drugs) have been used, but only very few of them have been studied for safety in pregnancy. Those that have been studied generally have a somewhat low grade of safety, so their use is discouraged unless the situation is dire. These should only be used under the direction of a veterinarian.

Antibiotics should generally be used during pregnancy only if absolutely necessary. A very small number of antibiotics are listed as safe for developing embryos. In general amoxicillin and ampicillin (both penicillin derivatives) are safe and are labelled as category A drugs. Both drugs cross the placenta and the mammary glands, so they easily become available to fetuses or puppies. All other antibiotics should be used with caution and only after consulting a reproductive safety study or statement.

Routine deworming medications, including heartworm preventative medicine, are known to be safe in pregnancy and do not need to be withdrawn during pregnancy. The drug classes that are known to be safe include ivermectin, pyrantel, fenbendazole, milbemycin oxime and selamectin.

Flea and tick preventions should be examined carefully. The isoxazoline-substituted benzamide derivatives such as spinosad, afoxolaner, sarolaner, and fluralaner have had adverse results in safety studies and should be avoided. Be sure to read package inserts carefully because these drugs are in multiple formulations that are commonly used. Use of preventatives has become the standard of care for most dogs, and withdrawing the use of them can put the brood bitch at risk of contracting diseases that these ectoparasites may carry. Reducing their use can also potentially increase parasitic load within her body. Breeders can switch to a product that is safe for pregnancy and lactation prior to mating to ensure safe transition and uninterrupted coverage during a pregnancy.

10.6 Disorders of Pregnancy

Bitches generally have very few problems during pregnancy. All goes well provided that the breeder provides adequate nutrition, a biosecure and safe environment in which to gestate, and avoids excess supplementation with unnecessary foodstuffs. Any clinical disease can potentially have a negative effect on pregnancy. Fever or other systemic illness will alter the metabolic processes within her body and may change how she supports a growing litter. Avoiding any situation where she may be exposed to a disease is best.

During the second half of pregnancy the corpora lutea are supported by the hormone prolactin. There is a gradual drop in progesterone concentrations throughout this time in pregnancy. This is a healthy and normal occurrence. The specific level of progesterone in a pregnant bitch can vary from animal to animal and pregnancy to pregnancy. The level may or may not be considered as normal depending on the interaction of the stage of pregnancy, the individual animal, and the individual pregnancy.

Despite the lack of a specific cutoff level, deficiency of adequate progesterone is one potential problem in maintaining a pregnancy. This can be either primary or secondary. Primary low progesterone occurs in a few animals that have an inadequate ability to produce this essential hormone. Low function of corpora lutea (primary hypoluteism or primary low progesterone) is very rare and can only be diagnosed with careful examination and testing by a veterinarian to rule out any systemic causes. Ruling out other causes can help to arrive at a diagnosis of primary hypoluteism.

Secondary low progesterone can occur because many diseases cause a release of prostaglandins because of the inflammation that they produce. Prostaglandins can negatively affect the corpora lutea that produce progesterone and maintains the pregnancy. This effect on the corpora lutea and the subsequent fall in progesterone can easily be confused with the primary sort of progesterone insufficiency, leading owners to think that the affected bitch is inherently unable to maintain a sufficient level of progesterone. It is important to distinguish between this primary low progesterone and a low progesterone that may be secondary to a natural response to systemic inflammation, because the two sorts have different needs for clinical support and management.

Low progesterone in middle to late gestation, for any reason, needs to be approached with extreme caution. Supplementation with progesterone brings with it potential risks and should be undertaken very cautiously. One risk is that bitches cannot whelp while under the influence of progesterone, so any supplementation needs to be withdrawn 2 to 3 days prior to the expected day of whelping. A further risk is that bitches supplemented with progesterone have low levels of milk production (hypogalatorrhea) and may have inadequate milk for the litter. The breeder needs to consider why progesterone is low, how important it is to supplement progesterone in the specific individual case, and if such treatment is wise if it is furthering a bloodline that can only successfully maintain a pregnancy if progesterone is supplemented externally.

Pregnancy toxemia is a condition that can occur in the last few weeks of pregnancy. This condition is due to an overall negative energy balance and can lead to very severe systemic disease. It is generally seen in bitches in a poor plane of nutrition (Figure 10.6). In pregnancy toxemia the bitches diet and body can no longer support the pregnancy. The result can be

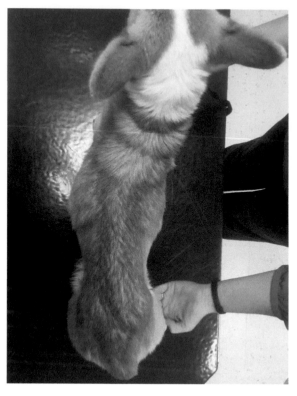

Figure 10.6 This bitch developed pregnancy toxemia, and then required significant assistance in whelping and was unable to raise her litter. The poor body condition is dramatic in this post-whelping photo but was not readily apparent when she was pregnant. The poor body condition is the underlying factor in this case of pregnancy toxemia. Photo by JTC.

a generalized wasting of body condition associated with anorexia, vomiting, and diarrhea. The two most common causes are:

- feed that is not formulated for pregnancy
- a few days of not eating
- a few days of vomiting.

Many bitches will have some degree of decreased appetite during the last 2 to 3 weeks of gestation. This is due to the rapidly increasing size of her uterus, causing it to take up more and more of the space in her abdomen. She will start using up her own fat and muscle to support the litter if she is unable to consume the needed calories to support the rapid growth of the puppies in late gestation. If this situation is not diagnosed and treated quickly, the whole litter (and possibly the bitch) may be lost to the downward spiral of the bitch beginning to sacrifice her own body tissues to maintain the pregnancy. Any changes in feed consumption by a late-gestation bitch should be considered seriously.

Breeders should be sure that the brood bitch is consuming adequate amounts of a balanced diet that will support pregnancy. Enticing her with table scraps and wet food may help, but sometimes force feeding is necessary to ensure that adequate caloric intake is occurring. Multiple small meals during a day can also be helpful in getting a bitch in late pregnancy to consume enough. Feed stuffs that are dense in calories, along with a well-balanced wet food, should be kept on hand for situations such as these. If a home-cooked approach is taken, be sure that it is balanced and recognize that most of these diets do not provide adequate nutrition. Seek help from a veterinary nutritionist.

Rapid distension of the abdomen in late gestation warrants veterinary examination. One cause of this is a condition similar to the hydrops condition that occurs in large animals. This is an emergency as it is a rapid accumulation of fluid within the uterus and can lead to difficulty maintaining normal systemic blood pressure. Dogs in late gestation that have a large change in the shape of the abdomen, and that are lethargic, or weak, should be examined immediately.

Bitches that have any major abrupt increase in water intake and urine output should be examined promptly, because this can be a sign of gestational diabetes. This is a rare condition that only occasionally occurs in dogs. It can have significant effects on both the dam and the litter. Most bitches affected with gestational diabetes are middle-aged and in the second half of gestation. Many hormones associated with pregnancy also influence insulin resistance, which makes regulation of glucose levels very difficult in affected bitches. The regulation of blood glucose in these animals is quite difficult, and in some cases is only possible after the abortion of the litter. In some cases, this can return the dam's glucose metabolism back to normal and prevent her death. Not all the bitches affected with gestational diabetes will be able to normalize blood glucose even after the litter is aborted or born, so extreme care is warranted when this disease occurs.

On the rare occasion that a pregnant bitch requires sedation or anesthesia, knowing when and how to safely perform the procedure is necessary. A pregnant bitch can metabolize drugs without much assistance and with little to no risk to the puppies, although this does depend on the specific drug(s) used. It is important to consider the procedure that needs to be done, the minimal drug use and dosage required to perform the procedure adequately, and the amounts of drug needed for full pain control. The main consideration of consistent uterine perfusion is key to ensure that the puppies are getting sufficient oxygen and nutrient exchange during the procedure.

Mid-pregnancy is the safest window of time for any elective procedure that is time sensitive and cannot be delayed. This time window avoids the early embryonic stage of development that occurs prior to pregnancy diagnosis and avoids the last trimester when the abdomen is enlarged, and perfusion of the uterus becomes more difficult. The options of sedation or anesthesia should be considered carefully and consultation with a veterinarian undertaken to ensure the best possible outcome, even if this means deciding that the bitch is more important than the puppies at any given stage of gestation.

10.7 Elective Termination of Pregnancy

Occasionally the termination of a pregnancy is desired. Most often this occurs due to an error in which the wrong male has mated a bitch for some reason or another. In most instances this error is caught soon after the mating. Other situations for pregnancy termination include severe systemic illness that develops in a pregnant bitch. This sort of situation can occur at any time during a pregnancy. The protocols for termination of a pregnancy vary depending on the specific time interval following mating, and on the availability of the required drugs from country to country.

One extreme method is surgical removal of the uterus. This is only realistic if the female is no longer intended for use in the breeding program. It is also a top choice for situations with hydrops of the pregnant uterus or other disorders of pregnancy.

During the first trimester it is possible to disrupt the pregnancy by using drugs that are antagonistic to the progesterone receptors. These are not currently licensed for use in the USA but are available in other countries.

After mid-gestation, a pregnancy can be terminated either with prostaglandins to lyse the corpora lutea, or with products that antagonize prolactin, or with antagonists to the progesterone receptors.

A common practice historically was the use of synthetic long-acting estrogens within a few days following a mismating. Estrogen delayed the passage of embryos into the uterus, leading to their demise. This was very successful in most cases, despite prolonging the clinical standing estrus for weeks. The use of synthetic estrogens can cause other systemic problems over time, and therefore their use should be restricted. In some cases, they can cause the bitch to cease the production of blood cells, which ultimately leads to her death.

Pregnancy termination, by whatever means, is accompanied by risks to the bitch's health and well-being. It should therefore never be used as a routine practice for controlling canine reproduction. Surgery is always to be taken seriously. Prostaglandins can cause severe systemic reactions. These protocols should only be used rarely and for medical necessity, rather than as routine tools.

10.8 Key Points

- Biosecurity practices keep the pregnant bitch safe from infectious disease.
- Dietary supplements must be used with care.
- Appropriate exercise is an important part of pregnancy management.
- Pregnancy diagnosis is important after mating, and can be done by ultrasound, palpation, measurement of relaxin, or radiography.
- Pregnant bitches should be strategically dewormed.
- Drugs and other pharmaceuticals should be avoided, and when this is not possible the drugs should be checked for their safety rating.
- Disorders of pregnancy are rare but important when they occur and may include:
  - o deficiency of progesterone
  - o pregnancy toxemia
  - o hydrops
  - o gestational diabetes mellitus.
- Protocols for pregnancy termination do exist, but each of them comes with risks.

CHAPTER 11

Whelping

The culmination of a successful mating is the birth of the puppies. The general term for this is "parturition" and for dogs the specific term is "whelping." The very active and dramatic events of whelping contrast with the relatively external calm of the previous two months of gestation. Whelping can cause high anxiety even for the most experienced breeder. A few strategic actions can be combined with a baseline of good husbandry and will adequately prepare for successful whelping. Consistently good husbandry throughout pregnancy always assures the highest rate of good outcomes at whelping, and a good basic recommendation is to always include exercise right up to the last few days of pregnancy prior to birth.

Preparation for whelping is important. Understanding the normal whelping process can help the breeder to quickly recognize anything abnormal. This ensures that any deviation from normal can be dealt with early and successfully. It is best to have multiple plans in place to allow for quick intervention should any adverse event arise.

Preparation for the whelping should occur well in advance of the expected date and should include plans for what to do in an emergency.

- Involve a veterinarian in the process from the very beginning.
- Be sure to have the whelping room ready well in advance.
- Stock the nutrition room with wet food and with milk replacer.
- Prepare for the possibility of a nervous bitch.
- When appropriate, have a few extra hands available, ideally someone that is already familiar to the bitch. The availability of extra help assures that even if the usual caretaker is absent during a whelping, someone else will be on site to assist.

11.1 Gestational Length

The estrous cycle and gestation of the bitch have unique aspects that unfortunately make prediction of a precise due date very challenging (Figure 11.1).

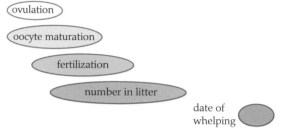

Figure 11.1 Several factors contribute to the variability of gestational length in dogs. Despite the difficulty of pinpointing whelping, it is sure that it will occur over a reasonably short number of hours when it finally arrives! Figure by DPS.

Dates on which matings occurred are unreliable predictors of a whelping date. Several factors contribute to uncertainty as to the exact moment of conception and initiation of pregnancy:

- the day of ovulation can be difficult to define
- the rate at which oocytes mature after ovulation can vary
- semen remains viable in the female reproductive tract for multiple days so that conception can occur over a range of a few days rather than just one.

These three factors combine to produce a window for fertilization that is several days long. It is impossible to determine a consistently accurate gestational length in the absence of an ovulation date. Ovulation is most accurately related to the date of the peak of luteinizing hormone, but is more practically pinpointed by the date of the progesterone surge or the date of cytologic diestrual shift.

Estimates for gestational length have been derived from the length of time between natural mating independent of any luteinizing hormone or progesterone timing. This estimate varies from 53 to 72 days. Relying on this long window of time is risky for anticipating whelping and is especially poor for scheduling caesarian sections. Puppies' lungs mature only in the final 24 to 48 hours of gestation, and if they are taken from the uterine environment before this they will fail to thrive and most often expire within days of being born. This makes accurate timing for a caesarian section essential.

Wise breeders accurately time the mating of dogs by documenting the day of ovulation, which can be done by monitoring progesterone levels. An alternative is to use daily vaginal cytology to try to pinpoint the diestrual shift. Cytology is also useful in situations where progesterone levels have been measured but for some reason have already elevated to post-ovulation levels, thereby failing to document the precise day of ovulation.

Each different method that determines the date of ovulation can be used to predict gestational length, but unfortunately each yields a different number of days. This is because each of them has a different relationship to the actual time of ovulation. The gestational length that is calculated from the peak in luteinizing hormone is around 65 days. The length from the actual date of ovulation is around 63 days. The length from the cytologic diestrual shift is around 57 days. Each of these estimates has a range that is one to two days longer or shorter. They each vary depending on the accuracy of the method used to time these events along with other factors.

Litter size is an important factor influencing gestational length. Litters with more puppies are carried for a shorter time than litters with fewer puppies. Another source of variability is the breed of dog. Some breeds of dogs are known to have shorter gestation lengths. These include Cavalier King Charles Spaniels, Bernese Mountain Dogs, and perhaps a few others. Within nearly all breeds, some genetic lines have short gestational lengths when compared to the breed average. Owners benefit by keeping good records of dates for ovulation and whelping so that they and their veterinarian are well aware of the animals that deviate from the averages.

A few methods can help to narrow down a whelping date, even if no timing was performed during the actual mating or no diestrual shift was identified on serial vaginal cytology of the bitch during estrus. Gestational aging can be accomplished by ultrasound about mid-gestation, or 30 days from the mating. An experienced vet-erinarian can measure specific fetal structures at this time to provide an accurate due date within a range of about 48 hours. Delaying this measurement until after 40 days of gestation makes it more cumbersome and less accurate, especially for brachyce-phalic breeds of dogs.

Another method to predict a whelping date relies on "reverse progesterone timing." This can be used in situations where other methods have not been performed and can accurately predict when stage one labor is likely to occur. The use of this technique is based on the fact that progesterone must be maintained at or above a level of 2 ng/ml for a pregnancy to remain in the uterus. A drop in progesterone below 2 ng/ml indicates that labor should begin within 24 hours. This can be tracked with a progesterone analyte machine and is reliable in most situations. Some pregnancies with only a single puppy may not produce enough signal to lyse the corpus luteum, and consequently the progesterone level will not drop.

An important detail is that progesterone levels drop very rapidly right before whelping. This drop can occasionally occur after a sample is taken, and in this situation the sample will have missed the drop. Despite this drawback, the technique is useful for animals that have a completely unknown ovulation date or cytologic shift. This method requires daily progesterone blood samples and careful interpretation and is usually combined with fetal ultrasound which can demonstrate maturity of the fetal kidney and gastrointestinal tract. However, ultrasound can be misleading if used alone to determine fetal maturity, so it should always be combined with progesterone levels or some other form of timing for the highest likelihood of live and vigorous puppies.

A drop in body temperature is another measurement that has been used widely by breeders and veterinarians alike. Progesterone is thermogenic, so when it is present the bitch's temperature rises. When progesterone levels fall below 2 ng/ml there is a transient drop in temperature (approximately 1°C or 2°F), well into the 36.6°C (98°F) range in con-trast to the usual canine body temperature of 37.5°C or 100.5°F. Once body temperature drops, labor is expected to begin within 24 hours. However, not all temperature drops are recognized, nor do all bitches have a temperature drop. Placement of the thermometer is important, as insertion into feces may incorrectly result in a very low temperature. When there is any doubt in the accuracy of the measurement, recheck the temperature after the bitch has defecated. The temperature should be checked at the same time(s) every day, following a consistent routine.

11.2 Selecting Natural Birth or Scheduled Caesarian Section

Whelping can occur in a few different ways, each of which has risks and benefits (Figure 11.2). The goal of both breeder and veterinarian is to have the best outcome possible for the dam and her offspring. The best outcomes in most instances are assured by avoiding the need for any medical or surgical management of a whelping. The need for these interventions most commonly arises from dystocia (difficult birth) or other abnormalities of parturition. A first step in avoiding problems is to select breeding stock that is known to be able to whelp on its own. Selecting and mating dogs with the goal of easy parturitions is an important contribution to successful whelping.

Some problems of parturition, such as primary uterine inertia (failure of uterine contractions) are rare. Breeders can avoid this problem even further by selecting for bitches that work hard in labor and produce puppies without being complacent. Bitches should be kept in good physical shape during the pregnancy because this prepares them for the work that labor requires. She should be fit enough to endure at least two to four hours of hard work that are involved in most whelpings.

Some specific dog breeds may require surgical delivery of puppies, although this can be avoided within even those breeds when breeders select a moderate physical type of dog that does not have a mismatch between the size of the fetal cranium and the maternal pelvic canal. It is wisest to avoid the routine use of elective caesarean sections (c-sections), because relying on this as a routine practice makes it impossible to identify and select bitches that can whelp naturally without assistance.

For those females that require a c-section it is best to set a limit of three elective abdominal procedures (including c-section or any others) over the life of the animal. Every incision into the abdomen comes with a risk of adhesion formation and scarring. These can

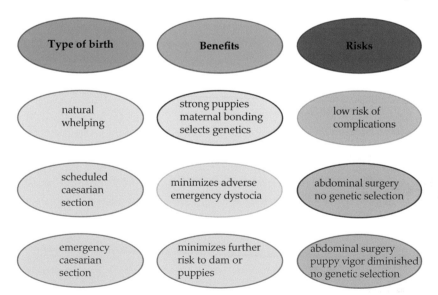

Figure 11.2 The different approaches to whelping have different risks for the dam, the puppies, and the breed. Figure by DPS.

lead to complications in non-reproductive organs (usually the intestinal tract) or adhesion formation between the uterus and other organs within the abdomen. Surgery should be a final option when adverse events indicate that it is appropriate. It should not be a routine elective choice. Surgery needs to be taken very seriously and should be avoided whenever possible.

If it is anticipated that a bitch will require a c-section, accurate timing of mating and conception should always be performed at the beginning of the pregnancy to narrow down a reasonably accurate time window for delivery. On the day scheduled for a c-section, the veterinarian should perform an ultrasound exam to check for signs of fetal maturity prior to surgery. This also serves as an opportunity to examine the fetuses and can help to avoid surprises such as discovering an abnormality of one or more of the puppies.

11.3 The Whelping Room

Breeders need to prepare several things in advance of the whelping. The design and furnishing of the actual whelping area should be considered around the time of pregnancy diagnosis. A whelping area should be outside of the general flow of a house or kennel, free from drafts, and have temperature and humidity that are easily controlled. Environmental control is important because puppies have a high content of water in their bodies and cannot maintain their own body temperature for the first three weeks of life.

Bitches prefer to whelp in a den-like area, tightly enclosed and dark. This aspect should be considered when planning a whelping area. Breeders can select from among many commercially available whelping boxes. Any whelping area should have easy access for a bitch while not allowing the puppies to exit the area without a considerable amount of intentional climbing. Design of the entrance or exit should take into consideration the pendulous aspect of the bitch's mammary chain during lactation. This helps to avoid trauma to her as she enters and exits the box (Figure 11.3).

A "pig rail" along the sides of the whelping box serves as a protected outlet for puppies and allows them to easily make an escape away from the bitch when she lies down.

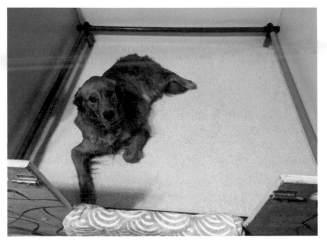

Figure 11.3 This is a well-designed whelping box with good textured flooring and a rail along the sides that allows the puppies to avoid being crushed by the bitch. Photo by Renee Machen.

This reduces the chance that she may accidentally crush or suffocate the puppies. The rail is offset towards the interior from the side of the box and provides a space below.

If a bitch continues to search for a more den-like atmosphere, the whelping box can be made more cave-like. It can be moved into a closet, or an exercise pen can be placed around the outside of the box and draped in dark sheets. These additions help the area to feel more like the environment of a secure den. Some bitches prefer to whelp in a kennel with solid walls. A crate that has a removable top is ideal for this purpose, because once she starts whelping it is possible to remove the top for better observation and to provide access for any necessary intervention. After whelping the bitch and her litter can be transferred from the crate into a whelping box.

Bedding for the whelping box should be disposable or easily washed. It should also have a varied texture. Any shavings that are used should be free of dyes or scents as these can be irritating to the dam and puppies. Varied texture, especially bedding and flooring that is not too smooth or slick, will help the puppies move around in the box and will prevent "swimmer puppy syndrome." Choice of a specific bedding option needs to consider whether a specific female is an excessive nester. Bitches with an excess of nesting behavior sometimes destroy any bedding that is put into the whelping area. Some bitches may actually shred the material by chewing it, and some bitches will then ingest it. Be prepared to remove the bedding if she is eating it. Ingestion of foreign bodies at this point is very detrimental to her health and health management.

It is ideal to start acclimating the bitch to the whelping area once the whelping box is set up. A good way to accomplish this is to start feeding her in the box one to two weeks prior to whelping. She will then associate the area with a positive experience. She should also sleep there at night.

Whelping is a drastic change in the daily routine of a bitch, especially for those that tend to be nervous or those that are accustomed to a very active lifestyle routine. These bitches can benefit from having an Adaptil® diffuser in the whelping room. This product contains pheromones that help dogs to feel relaxed and comfortable. While not rigorously proven to be effective, the diffuser is not doing any harm and might indeed help, and it is therefore better to have this in the room prior to whelping rather than needing it after the bitch begins the whelping process.

11.4 Veterinary Roles

A positive working relationship between breeder and veterinarian can contribute to successful pregnancy and whelping. If the veterinarian has been involved since the mating it is likely that conversations have occurred about managing any potential dystocia. Breeders should have one or two alternate plans if the regular veterinarian is not available when the bitch is whelping. Ideally the veterinary practice that is identified has a facility that can perform ultrasound, bloodwork, and surgery during the day and afterhours, seven days a week. If these services are not available, the breeder should arrange with their regular veterinarian to identify a clinic that can provide support if a problem arises outside of normal working hours. This should be done well in advance of the bitch's due date.

It may be difficult to find a clinic that is available or willing to see a dystocia as an emergency in situations where a bitch was mated and managed only by the breeder and has not had any follow up care during the pregnancy. Long-term client-patient-veterinarian relationships are well-advised. An additional reason for this is that the veterinarian is required for the dispensing of any prescribed medications. Bitches should only be administered drugs under the guidance of a veterinarian, so it is always best to have an ongoing relationship with them.

11.4.1 Pre-Whelping Radiographs

One useful veterinary procedure is a pre-whelping radiograph, which is helpful in a number of ways (Figure 11.4). For bitches that will be free whelping, it is best to know the litter size that can be expected. This allows the breeder time to prepare, to double check their wait list, and can also help in making decisions if a problem should arise during whelping. The information revealed by the radiograph is necessary for the veterinarian to offer appropriate options during a dystocia. The decision tree may be altered drastically depending on whether a bitch in trouble has three to five puppies remaining, versus only one or two. The breeder also may approach decisions regarding dystocia management differently depending on the radiograph. A team-based approach between the veterinarian and breeder, combined with fetal numbers and other diagnostics, will make this process move forward practically and quickly.

Radiographs are routinely performed approximately one week prior to the bitch's due date. This requires one or two lateral views with the bitch lying on her side. In litters with eight puppies or fewer the fetal count is usually straightforward as the puppies are spread out and easily counted by following skulls and spines. When there are more than eight puppies the counting can become quite difficult. In that situation, good radiographic technique and experience are both helpful. In addition to information on the number of expected fetuses, a radiograph allows for one more veterinary examination close to the time of whelping. This is a time to discuss many topics including how to determine if there is a problem in whelping, what to do when a problem arises, and whom to call in

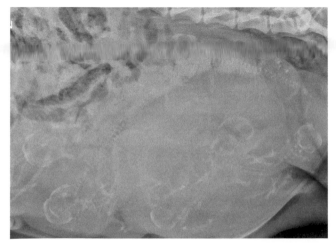

Figure 11.4 A pre-whelping radiograph gives important information about the number and development of the puppies. Photo by JTC.

the event of a dystocia. Nutritional adjustments and other late-pregnancy issues can also be discussed.

It is generally not routine to radiograph animals that are certain to require a caesarean section, because all of the fetuses will be easily found and can be removed during the surgery without a count beforehand. This level of care is currently debated, though, because radiographs can minimize the chances of missing a puppy during a caesarian section.

11.5 *Events in Whelping*

The actual whelping is a very complex cascade of events that occurs over two to four days and includes the shorter time span of the actual expulsion of the puppies. Many hormones participate in whelping. Each of them has its own specific role and has important interactions with the others. The details of some of the interactions have yet to be documented.

Once the fetuses mature, they begin to release the stress hormone cortisol, which then causes a down-stream release of other hormones. The hormonal signals increase the numbers of receptors for oxytocin and relaxin so that the body is more responsive to these. Cortisol also directly enhances the production of prostaglandins, resulting in the release of several forms of prostaglandin by the bitch. The prostaglandins are an important trigger, because they result in complete lysis (death) of the corpora lutea over a span of about 24 to 36 hours. The sudden demise of the corpora lutea causes a drop in progesterone levels, with the result that the ratio of circulating progesterone and estrogen concentrations becomes inverted from the ratio present during gestation. Prostaglandins also relax the cervix which helps to assure easy passage of the puppies during parturition. Oxytocin is another essential hormone in whelping because it aids in uterine contraction. Relaxin contributes to successful whelping by causing relaxation of the connective tissues of the pelvis and cervix to ensure the largest diameter possible for the birth canal. Prolactin also contributes and is prominent in the second half of gestation by supporting the function of corpora lutea up until they are lysed. Prolactin peaks a bit later than some of the other hormones, with the peak occurring during lactation to help support milk production. The entire hormonal concert must be intact for parturition to begin and terminate normally.

Parturition is divided into three distinct phases in domestic animals, commonly referred to as stages one through three (Figure 11.5). Each stage has normal parameters that breeders should be noting during whelping. Each stage also has a few potential markers of concern that indicate when to seek veterinary assistance.

Stage one is characterized by nesting, hyporexia (decreased appetite) or anorexia (no appetite), restlessness, panting and seeking out dark places to hide. This stage corresponds with an increase in uterine contractions and dilation of the cervix, but no active pushing occurs in stage one. Stage one should begin within 24 hours of a temperature drop (if one was detected) and can last for up to 12 to 18 hours. Bitches may nest off and on for several days prior to true stage one labor, but these sessions generally occur infrequently and for only a few minutes each time. Vulvar discharge at this time will likely be clear mucus with no color. Frequent small meals can be offered in stage one, as well as water or electrolyte solution. Walking a bitch during this time is also helpful to allow her to eliminate any urine in her bladder. Walking also helps to stimulate uterine contractions.

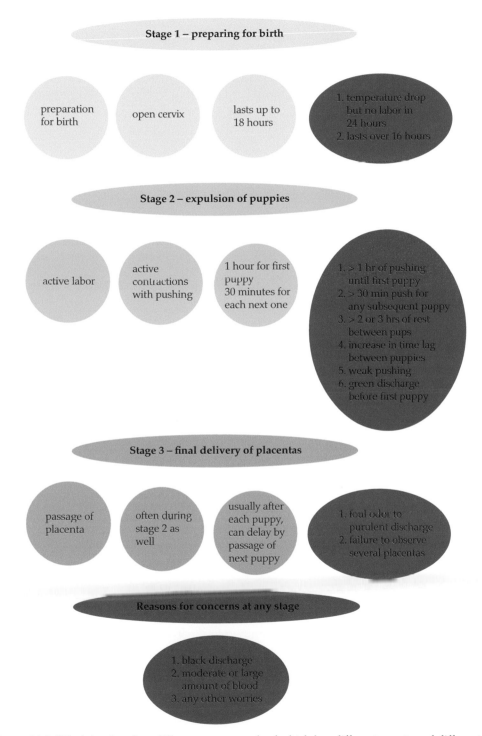

Figure 11.5 Whelping involves different stages, each of which has different events and different signals for alarm and intervention. Figure by JTC.

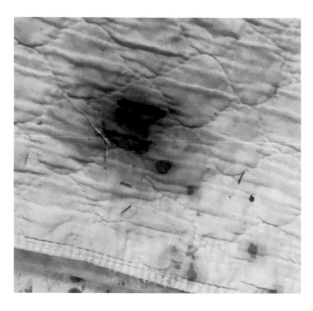

Figure 11.6 The green discharge that accompanies whelping can be alarming to novices but is completely normal. Photo by JTC.

If the bitch does not progress into stage two labor by 18 hours a veterinarian should examine her. Ultrasound can help in this situation and is the only imaging modality that will be able to give reliable fetal heart rates, determine quality and quantity of fetal movement, and identify any abnormalities in puppies.

Stage two is the active portion of labor and is characterized by forceful uterine contractions along with pushing by the bitch. Bitches should bear down and give strong abdominal pushes that help to expel puppies. Some bitches are very overt in their pushing, while others may only have a pause in their panting coupled with a quick but forceful push. Normal vulvar discharges vary from clear fluid, serosanguinous (red-tinged), or green. The green discharge is known as uteroverdin. It can be surprising but is normal and derives from the material at the margins of the placentas. Uteroverdin is a consequence of normal placental detachment in dogs (Figure 11.6).

Puppies are normally produced at intervals of no longer than 30 minutes to an hour. The probability of a stillborn puppy increases in situations when this time interval is longer. Offering food and or water during stage two is fine, but the bitch should not be forced to eat or drink. Allowing her to eat the placentas provides an energy source and fosters normal maternal behaviour. She should be allowed to clean puppies and sever the umbilical cords on her own. A breeder can watch carefully but should allow the bitch the freedom to do what comes naturally. One common but unfounded fear is that an overly attentive bitch can cause umbilical hernias if she is too vigorous in attending to the placenta and umbilicus. Umbilical hernias do not result from excessive pulling by the bitch, but instead are a defect present at birth and not the result of the dam's actions. The same is true of other abdominal midline defects that sometimes are blamed on the dam's actions during whelping.

If dystocia is going to occur, it occurs in stage two. Dystocia rates in dogs vary from 2% to 23% of all births in bitches. Toy and brachycephalic breeds are more likely to experience dystocia than are other types of dogs. The frequency of dystocia increases with several risk factors:

- litters that have fewer than three to five puppies
- bitches that are older
- smaller bitches
- smaller breeds
- breeds with brachycephalic conformation.

The following are reasons that an owner should call the veterinarian or automatically present the bitch for an examination.

- Failure to produce the first puppy in one hour of stage two labor. The longer a bitch pushes unproductively, the more excess energy she expends. This also increases the risk of the remaining fetuses becoming stressed.
- Any time that she is actively pushing for more than 30 minutes to an hour for each subsequent puppy or takes a nap with no contractions for greater than three hours.
- Increasing intervals between puppies can indicate that a bitch is reaching exhaustion and is a sign of possible dystocia.
- If the amnion (inner placenta) of the puppy is visualized and a puppy is not produced within 30 minutes (Figure 11.7)
- The vulvar discharge is:
  o black
  o acutely hemorrhagic with frank blood (bright red)
  o green discharge for greater than 30 minutes with no puppy produced.

The risk of dystocia increases for bitches that have been anorexic for one to two days prior to the whelping and will then not eat during a whelping. The bitch's muscles require glucose for proper function, and food is the best source of this nutrient. Wet food can be more palatable than dry kibble and will encourage the reluctant bitch to eat. Sugar water or milk replacer can also be used. Some bitches will eat ice cream or yogurt, and these are great sources of energy. Some people mistakenly assume that

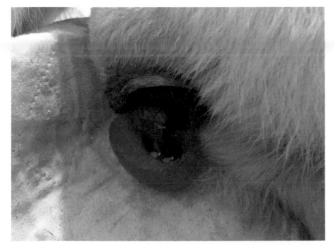

Figure 11.7 The amnion in this photo is protruding as a bubble from the vulva, and the puppy's feet and claws can be seen through the membrane. Photo by Kathy Marr.

ice cream or yogurt are also effective for quickly supplementing calcium, but this is not true. Supplementation or administration of anything other than food during a whelping should only be done under the guidance of a veterinarian as more harm than good may occur.

A number of procedures that have been used during whelping are of doubtful need or effectiveness and include.

- Calcium supplementation is thought to increase the strength of contractions but is controversial. No dietary form of calcium-containing product will provide enough calcium to have an appreciable effect on the body over the relatively short time frame of labor.
- Oxytocin administration increases the frequency of contractions but is potentially dangerous when not properly monitored.
- Tocodynametry is the tracking of uterine contraction waveforms obtained through an abdominal monitor. This is used in human medicine but has not been validated as useful in dogs and cannot replace the examination of the animal by a veterinarian.
- Fetal heart rate monitoring with a doppler unit must be interpreted cautiously. There are many large vessels within the abdomen of the bitch, and it is possible to detect the bitch's heart rate rather than a fetal heart rate.

The use of any pharmaceuticals during labor should only be used in concert with the careful fetal monitoring that is available within a veterinary practice. Use of pharmaceuticals increases the risk of stillbirths. When indicated, surgical intervention should be rapidly initiated. Delayed surgical intervention may be reserved for cases only after medical management has failed. This can result in a higher rate of stillborn puppies when compared to cases in which surgical management was used as a first choice when problems were first encountered. Having the bitch in a veterinary clinic setting provides for opportunities to closely examine the bitch and to monitor fetal distress in real time. This allows the opportunity to quickly change dystocia management from medical management to surgical management when necessary.

Stage three of parturition is the passage of the placenta. Each puppy has its own individual placenta. Most placentas are passed right after the puppy or even with the puppy, but normal passage can take up to thirty minutes after the puppy has passed through the birth canal. Retained placentas in the bitch are not a major cause of concern, except in cases when no placentas were seen during the entire whelping. If a large number of placentas are not accounted for during a whelping this should be communicated to the veterinarian so that they can assist in determining if treatment is necessary. It is best to allow the bitch to eat the placentas. This is natural behavior, and they are a source of energy for a bitch that might not otherwise be eating. Consumption of placentas can also contribute to maternal behavior.

11.6 A Pause in Whelping

Some bitches may have a pause while producing a litter with a moderate or large number of puppies. During this pause the bitch may clean and nurse her puppies or even take a nap. The nursing puppies produce a profound release of oxytocin, and they should be allowed to nurse as much as they will. If the bitch has been resting for greater than two hours, it is best that she gets up and goes outside for a brisk walk or even trot around the yard. This will stimulate contractions and hopefully jumpstart production of puppies within the next 15–30 minutes. She can be offered food and water during a pause.

11.7 When a Puppy Arrives

The hardest part of being a breeder is to patiently let nature take its course. Interfering with the natural progression of whelping can lead to prolonged labor and possible dystocia. When a bitch starts to whelp it is best to support from afar or just sit quietly and watch. Talking to or interacting with the bitch will only distract her from the job at hand. When the bitch delivers the first puppy let her clean and interact with the puppy and eat the placenta.

A few supplies are helpful during whelping and should be organized and available before the expected day arrives (Figure 11.8). These include a gram scale to weigh the puppy on, and a bowl or container to put the puppy in during weighing. Surgical gloves help to keep the attendant free of birth fluids and minimize the contamination of the dam or puppy during whelping. A good obstetrical lubricant can be useful if the bitch needs assistance in passing a puppy through the birth canal. A hemostat can be used to clamp an umbilical cord that is bleeding excessively, and dental floss or suture can be used to tie it off. Colored yarn can be used as a loose collar to identify puppies that are similar in color and sex. Bulb syringes are handy if excess mucus needs to be removed from a puppy's airway. Bandage scissors can help if any of these other supplies need to be cut safely.

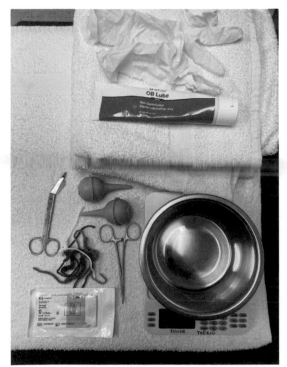

Figure 11.8 A useful array of whelping supplies include gloves, lubricant, bulb syringe, hemostat, scissors, suture, puppy identification collars, a scale, and a bowl or other utensil to weigh the puppy in. Photo by JTC.

The history of the management practices at one working kennel is instructive. The kennel requested veterinary help because it had a high rate of dystocias. The kennel had instituted a practice of routinely feeding the whelping bitches after the production of each puppy. During this time, the attendants carefully cleaned and weighed each puppy. The unintended consequence of this protocol was that the bitches learned to diligently beg for food rather than focusing on labor or nursing the puppies that had already been born. Following suggestions, the kennel switched to a management style that was more passive, observing labor remotely via camera. Personnel only entered the whelping room when trouble was evident, or after the dam had had time to clean the puppy on her own. After instituting this more relaxed management, the dystocia rates quickly fell to within the normal range.

If a puppy is born and is not vigorous or breathing, the first strategy is to let the dam attempt to revive it herself. If she needs assistance after a minute or so, stimulate respiration by rubbing the puppy with a clean, dry towel, clearing the airway with a bulb syringe and tugging on the umbilicus. A warm environment in which to whelp and recover puppies is always helpful in these situations. Some puppies will be "fish breathing" which is taking a large breath occasionally. Such a puppy is trying to come around and should continue to be rubbed vigorously. Pulling on the umbilicus also helps these puppies. The addition of mild warm heat will also help dry the puppy and will keep it warm until it is breathing more regularly. Slinging puppies to stimulate breathing should never be done because it causes intracranial damage to the brain.

Once the puppy is dry it is a good time to check its sex and for any birth defects, such as cleft palate, limb deformities, or other abnormalities (Figure 11.9). This is also the time to

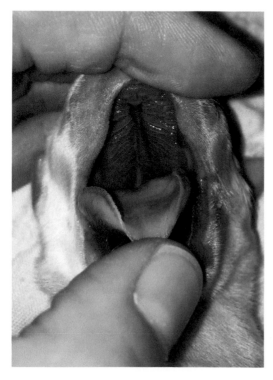

Figure 11.9 Cleft palate is one of the more common defects in newborns, leading to aspiration of milk into the lungs. Photo by JTC.

weigh the puppy with a gram or food scale. Weight gain is a reliable and easy indicator of health in neonates. Checking a birth weight prior to nursing allows a breeder to keep track of daily weight gain. Most normal puppies will nurse within 30 minutes to an hour after being born. A plateau or loss in weight over a 24-hour period is a clear indication of possible problems. Having the birth weight recorded from the outset is important.

Do not routinely tie off any umbilical cords. The crushing caused during the dam's active separation of the puppy from the placenta should cause adequate control of any bleeding. If bleeding continues to occur it can be controlled by tying off the umbilicus using sterile suture or non-waxed, non-flavored dental floss. A simple knot can be tied around the cord, with the ends of the thread cut very short.

A puppy born with any internal organs on the outside of the body presents a true emergency (Figure 11.10). A bitch can inadvertently sever the gastrointestinal tract of a puppy that has an abdominal midline defect through which the abdominal organs have prolapsed to the outside. Gently and cleanly pick the puppy up and present it to a veterinarian for examination. Surgery is not ideal in newborns as they do not possess normal blood clotting factors so significant hemorrhage is a risk. Anesthesia is very risky in newborn puppies. If any of the organs were damaged, humane euthanasia may be the best course of action for the puppy.

The rate of stillbirths increases with the length of whelping and the size of the litter. If a puppy is born that has a normal appearance yet is grey and non-responsive it is likely stillborn. If a puppy is born with black fluid or tissue surrounding it or has skin or hair that is sloughing this puppy has been dead in the uterus for a while and needs to be removed

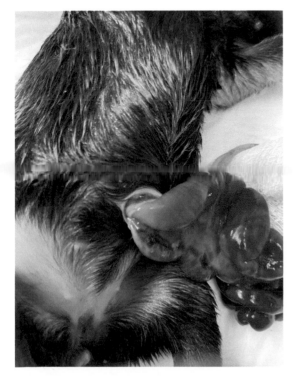

Figure 11.10 Some midline defects are mild, resulting in small umbilical hernias. In more severe cases the intestines can prolapse through the defect leading to death of the puppy. Photo by JTC.

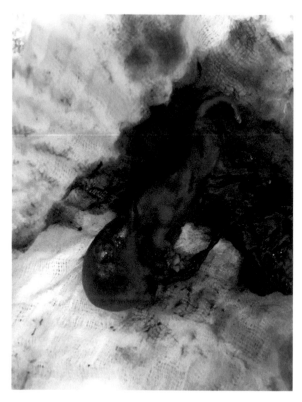

Figure 11.11 This puppy's condition of degeneration indicates that it has been dead in the uterus for some time. Photo by JTC.

immediately (Figure 11.11). The veterinarian should be informed of any puppies born in either of these conditions. The veterinarian can then advise on the best course of action.

Anasarca puppies, also known as water or walrus babies, are seen on occasion, and are more common in brachycephalic breeds than in other breeds (Figure 11.12). These puppies have an abnormal amount of fluid that is retained within the body and come out of the birth canal looking very round and having a jelly-like texture. The survival of these puppies depends on the severity of the condition, and they should be examined by a veterinarian immediately. There is a hereditary tendency for this condition and future breeding should be carefully considered for dams or sires that have produced an anasarca puppy.

11.8 Puppy Rejection

There are several reasons a bitch may reject a puppy or an entire litter. Strategies for an entire litter are different than those for a single rejected puppy. Maiden or nervous bitches will sometimes be confused or anxious after the delivery of the first few puppies. These bitches benefit from a calm environment and calm owners. Calming the bitch can also be aided with the Adaptil® diffuser. Many bitches that have a relatively low level of rejection behavior or that are overtly nervous after the first puppy is produced, may allow the handler to move her into a lateral position and then will allow the puppy(s) to nurse. This can help to get her to accept the puppies due to the release of oxytocin and other stimulation.

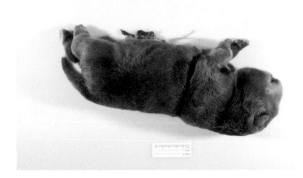

Figure 11.12 Puppies with anasarca are more common in some breeds than in others. The extra retention of fluid is especially noted on the head. Photo by T.E. Cecere.

Lactation and nursing rely on hormonal support. Nursing the puppies helps to induce maternal behavior and caring for puppies due to its interaction with oxytocin and other hormones (Figure 11.13). Nursing releases oxytocin, which has a natural calming effect on the bitch and contributes directly to maternal behavior. Scolding the bitch rarely contributes to enhancing the calm and accepting behavior that is needed. Likewise, removing a puppy from the bitch should be avoided unless she is going to hurt the puppy or owner. Some nervous bitches are calmed by using sepia, which is a natural remedy that is derived from cuttlefish. It can supplement natural oxytocin release that occurs with nursing or stripping milk. Intranasal oxytocin has also been used successfully to calm nervous bitches. Any oxytocin or sepia should only be used under the supervision of a veterinarian.

A bitch that is mothering and caring for most of the litter but refuses to nurse or clean a specific puppy is a different situation than a bitch rejecting an entire litter. Many dams will reject a single puppy when there is something wrong with that puppy. Breeders should be very careful in this situation because some bitches, if repeatedly offered the puppy or made to interact with a rejected puppy, will kill the puppy outright. The puppy should be removed and examined by a veterinarian. Many dams can sense that there is something wrong with the single rejected puppy. Many puppies that are singled out like this end up fading and dying despite expert care.

Any bitch that has undergone a caesarian section should be monitored very closely for any sign of rejecting the puppies for the first 24–48 hours after surgery. General anesthesia

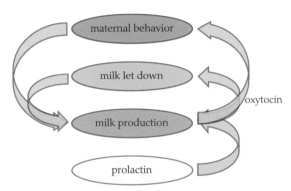

Figure 11.13 Milk production, milk let down, and maternal behavior can spark a feedback loop that enhances good outcomes for puppies and dams. Figure by DPS.

and other drugs administered during the procedure will alter her normal mentation. This will make her less aware of her surroundings, and some dams can have abnormal reactions during this time. These reactions are occasionally violent towards the puppies. For the highest chance of the best outcome for the dam and litter it is best to always have the owner present when the puppies are with their dam for the first few days after surgery. If no person is available to be with them for a period, the puppies should be removed during those times until the breeder is certain that the dam is mothering well and acting like her normal self. This is a short window of time for due diligence, and inattention during this period can end with a whole litter of severely traumatized or dead puppies.

11.9 *Key Points*

- Gestation length varies and is determined by day of ovulation, conception, and litter size.
- Whelping date can be estimated from ovulation date or other means such as:
  o progesterone surge at ovulation
  o cytologic changes at diestrus
  o palpation and fetal size mid-gestation
  o progesterone declines near whelping
  o body temperature drops near whelping.
- Routinely scheduled caesarian sections are generally to be avoided.
- A whelping room should be comfortable for the dam and the attendants.
- Pre-whelping radiographs can help to manage problems as they arise.
- Normal whelping has three stages:
  o stage 1 involving early contractions
  o stage 2 involving strong contractions and active pushing with birth of puppies
  o stage 3 involving the final passage of placentas.
- Dystocia outcomes are best when intervention is early.
- Puppy arrival should be managed by the bitch with minimal intervention.
- In the case of puppy rejection.
  o If an entire litter is rejected the bitch can be coaxed.
  o A single rejected puppy is likely abnormal and should be examined.

CHAPTER 12

Management in the Three Weeks Following Whelping

The three weeks following whelping are an important time for the bitch, for the litter, for breeders, and for breeding programs. During these three weeks the puppies undergo rapid growth and early developmental maturation, while the dam undergoes lactation and uterine involution. The breeder has important roles in managing both litter and dam during these few weeks, so a detailed understanding of postpartum care of the lactating dam and the growth of neonatal puppies helps to assure a good outcome. The goal during this period is to be able to avoid neonatal loss. The surest way to minimize loss is to identify problems quickly to manage appropriate interventions for the dam or the litter.

12.1 The Normal Post-Partum Dam

Management of the post-partum dam is essential to assure survival and growth of the puppies as well as the health and well-being of the dam. Knowing and recognizing the characteristics of a normal post-partum period can help to alert breeders to any deviations from normal so they can recognize when interventions may be helpful. As with most dog breeding, early intervention is always the most effective at correcting problems and ensuring good outcomes.

12.1.1 Uterine Involution and Normal Vulvar Discharge

The canine placenta is more invasive into the uterine wall than is typical of many other species. It can take up to two months after whelping to achieve full repair of the damage caused to the endometrial lining of the uterus because of this invasion. The fluid and remnants of tissue discarded during this process of repair exit through the vulva in the form of vulvar discharge. This discharge is called "lochia" in medical terminology and demonstrates several normal changes over the first three weeks following whelping. Immediately after whelping, the discharge is a thin fluid that is usually tinged with blood or can be brown. Over the next week to two weeks the discharge changes to mucoid in nature with a light brown or tan color. Some bitches have a vulvar discharge for up to 6 to 8 weeks post-partum. Vulvar discharge is a normal part of the resolution of the pregnancy during this period. The vulva and the discharge should be examined daily to monitor the progression of the involution process.

Signs of an abnormal process may include the following.

- A bitch with a fever.
- Discharge with a frank red color. Frank hemorrhage in excessive amounts, such as blood dripping from the vulva, warrants immediate examination.
- Discharge with a notably foul odor.

Two rare conditions in bitches result in overt bleeding of the endometrium, and blood will be expelled out of the vulva. These conditions are usually only treated when they involve a severe loss of blood that can be life threatening. The treatment is immediate surgical removal of the uterus along with blood transfusions to replace the blood that has been lost. These two conditions are.

- Subinvolution of placental sites (SIPS). This occurs when the invasive portion of the placentas is resolved either incompletely or is delayed. Most cases eventually resolve on their own, but this can take several weeks. When coupled with blood loss this can threaten the health of the bitch.
- Adenomyosis. This is a growth of uterine glands down into the muscle of the uterus. The invasion of the muscle tissue moves the endometrial glands closer to the external surface of the uterus, which increases the risk of penetration through this surface and into the body cavity.

12.1.2 Nutrition of the Lactating Bitch

While pregnancy is metabolically demanding, especially during the last few weeks, lactation is in fact the most nutritionally demanding stage of life for any bitch (Figure 12.1). Lactating bitches require consistent access to high-energy, high-quality diets. Their needs can be met by a food labelled for all life stages. Bitches that are raising large litters require thousands of calories a day, and this usually requires free choice feeding. The breeder should diligently measure the quantity of food the bitch is consuming to monitor her appetite and to be sure of adequate intake. Lactating bitches also require large amounts of water. Breeders need to prepare well in advance for the needs of the lactating bitch. It is best to have excess food on

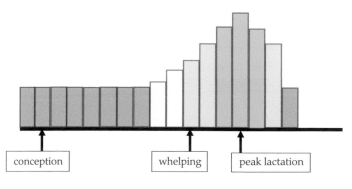

conception   whelping   peak lactation

Figure 12.1 Nutritional demands of a lactating bitch can be markedly higher than at any other time of her life. They rise slowly towards the end of gestation as the puppies enter their final growth spurt, and then peak rapidly after whelping and during lactation. Figure by DPS.

hand, and to be prepared to adjust the specific diet if the bitch has, or develops, any food aversions.

Peak lactation occurs between 2 to 3 weeks after parturition. This is the period during which the bitch requires the most caloric intake. Providing adequate nutrition is essential during early lactation to prevent any metabolic concerns that may arise in the post-partum period. Fortunately, after parturition the puppies no longer take up space in the bitch's abdomen, and no longer limit her stomach's capacity to hold food. A bitch that is overly fat or that has a small litter may not need as much food as those with less body fat or a larger litter. Bitches that are lean or have large litters become ravenous and caloric intake must be maintained. Close attention must be paid to body condition score, muscle condition score, and weight. It is always easier to put on weight on a dog than it is to take it off, and the food intake during the post-partum period can be adjusted quite easily.

12.2 Post-Partum Problems in Bitches

The most commonly encountered problems in the post-partum bitch include:

- hypogalactorrhea (poor lactation)
- mastitis (inflammation of the mammary gland, due to infection)
- hypocalcemia (low blood calcium leading to weakness)
- metritis (infection and inflammation of the uterus).

12.2.1 Hypogalactorrhea (Poor Lactation)

Bitches that do not have milk or colostrum at parturition are a concern for multiple reasons. The lack of milk available for puppies could be due to either one of two different processes – inadequate milk production, or some problem in the let-down of milk produced. Colostrum, or first milk, is different from the milk produced later in lactation. Colostrum contains valuable antibodies for puppies. Without these antibodies, the puppies are at risk for a wide range of infectious diseases. They are also at risk for inadequate nutrition.

Milk production is driven by the hormone prolactin. Milk production increases when the mammary gland is emptied of milk as the puppies nurse. Veterinarians can assist in boosting milk production with a few pharmaceuticals. Metoclopramide and domperidone are the two most commonly used drugs that can improve milk production. These are best used within the first 24 hours of lactation and should be used only in the doses that produce the desired effect.

Milk let-down is aided by the hormone oxytocin. Oxytocin can only produce milk let-down when there is actually milk within the gland. It will not assist in producing milk. The bitch's teats should be tested for the presence of milk a few times during the last day of pregnancy and the first day after whelping. After whelping the breeder should examine each mammary chain daily for any changes in milk consistency, such as a color change from white to purulent or bloody, along with any knots of firm tissue or areas of soreness.

12.2.2 Mastitis

Mastitis is one of the important conditions that can occur during lactation. This is inflammation within one or more mammary glands and is an indication of infection within the gland. Mastitis can occur early in lactation up through three to four weeks post-partum. Many bitches with mastitis will present with a swollen, hot mammary gland that may or may not have color changes within the skin (Figure 12.2). Some of these bitches will be off food and have a fever. Mastitis occurs in different frequencies in different genetic lines, which implies that at least some concern over a genetic influence is warranted.

When a case of mastitis is identified it needs to be treated immediately by a veterinarian. Medical treatment usually involves some combination of:

* antibiotics targeted at the bacteria found within the gland
* anti-inflammatory medications to reduce pain and swelling
* gastroprotectant medications to diminish any reluctance to eat.

One of the best ways to treat mastitis is to strip the milk out of the affected glands and this strategy should always be incorporated into the medical treatment plan. If the puppies are still nursing, it is wisest to continue to let them nurse. By doing this the puppies will not only be constantly emptying the gland of milk, but they will also be getting small doses of the antibiotics which can prevent problems if bacteria contaminate the milk. Puppies that are actively nursing are also indicating that the milk quality is still acceptable enough that there is no risk of milk toxicosis from ingestion of markedly changed or infected milk.

In situations where the puppies are not nursing ,the breeder then needs to strip the milk from the gland. This needs to be done multiple times a day. Warm and cold compresses alternately applied to the gland can relieve the pain associated with mastitis. Cabbage leaves can be chopped and laid against the affected gland. These have antibacterial properties as well as the ability to pull fluid out of tissues. Bitches usually become increasingly comfortable following a series of cabbage leaf compresses.

Gangrenous mastitis is a more severe disease process that involves death of portions of the gland (Figure 12.3). This is fairly rare and usually follows a milder initial bout of mastitis but is a serious condition that requires aggressive surgical debridement and open wound management by a veterinary professional. Treated appropriately, the dam will

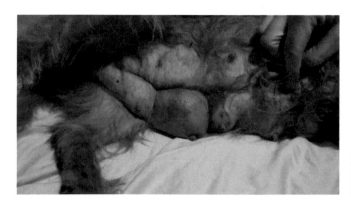

Figure 12.2 This mammary gland is swollen, hot, and discolored. Photo by Kara Kolster.

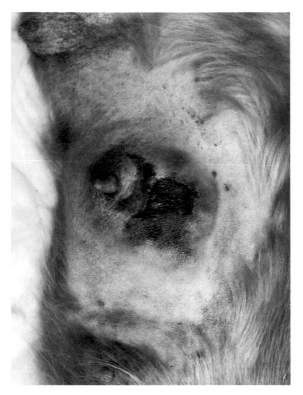

Figure 12.3 Gangrenous mastitis is often discolored due to death of mammary tissue. Photo by JTC.

recover, and any subsequent lactations will not be affected if the gland can be salvaged. Early detection and effective treatment are the keys to preventing long-term effects of gangrenous mastitis.

Bitches that have had mastitis once are prone to having it again in a subsequent lactation. This is best avoided by ensuring a very clean environment and diligence in checking mammary chains daily. Delay in treatment by as few as one or two days can adversely affect the outcome of treatment in the bitch. Delay not only affects the puppies because they may not gain weight appropriately during those days, but they are also being exposed to infected milk.

12.2.3 Hypocalcemia

Hypocalcemia is a condition that breeders justifiably dread. This condition is best avoided by ensuring proper nutrition during pregnancy and lactation. It is also avoided by eliminating any supplementation with calcium-containing products without direction by a veterinarian, even though this may seem counter-intuitive. Balanced commercial diets provide enough nutritional calcium to support lactation as long as the bitch is consuming adequate calories. Peak lactation, between two and three weeks post-partum, is the period of maximum demand for calcium.

Calcium is an essential nutrient because calcium levels in the blood must be maintained within narrow limits for muscle contraction to occur normally. This includes the heart muscle as well as skeletal muscle. Calcium levels are kept within the required limits by a balance of the dietary calcium that is coming into the dog and the dog's ability to mobilize calcium from bones and other tissue stores when incoming calcium is low. The control mechanisms interact in complex ways.

The risk of hypocalcemia in bitches increases with several factors:

- large litters
- inadequate food intake
- abrupt removal of calcium supplementation.

Bitches that have very large litters have a higher risk of developing hypocalcemia than those with smaller litters. This is due to the higher demand for milk that is imposed by all those puppies nursing, which stimulates the bitch to produce even more milk. Any bitches that are not eating, or are eating very little, need to be examined. This may be a sign that the bitch has a subclinical condition that needs treatment. Low food intake can lead to inadequate intake of calcium, forcing the bitch to mobilize the calcium stores from her bones to use these for milk production. Once her own stores are depleted, she will become hypocalcemic.

An important pathway to hypocalcemia is not particularly intuitive, at least superficially (Figure 12.4). Bitches that are fed calcium supplements and that are getting an abundance of calcium will inactivate the hormonal mechanism for drawing calcium out of the bone reserves because her diet is adequate (or more than adequate) at meeting her calcium requirements. The mechanism to mobilize calcium from bones is unfortunately not able to reactivate very quickly, and this can result in a temporary inability to maintain calcium levels in the normal range during a sudden peak in demand for calcium if the hormonal mechanism is inactive. Demand for calcium increases very rapidly at the beginning of lactation, and at this point it is difficult or impossible to meet the demand by dietary calcium alone, so the bitch depends on the ability to mobilize calcium from stores in the bone.

Therefore, it is best for the hormonal mechanisms that draw calcium from the bones to be up and effective at the time lactation begins. Supplementation during late gestation turns off those mechanisms and can never, or rarely, provide adequate calcium when the peak demand occurs. The result of supplementation is therefore a situation that nearly assures some level of transitory hypocalcemia. Unfortunately, the transitory nature of the condition can still be life-threatening due to the ongoing need for a tight balance of blood calcium levels to assure muscle function.

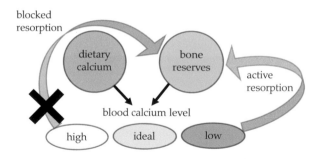

Figure 12.4 Control of blood calcium levels is essential for life, and abundant calcium supplementation can actually impede activation of control mechanisms. Figure by DPS.

Problems with calcium balance can result from home-cooked diets, which are often not balanced and most of which do not provide enough calcium to support the lactational demands. If these diets are fed over long periods of time the result can be the exhaustion of the bitch's ability to mobilize calcium, leading to hypocalcemia.

Clinical signs of hypocalcemia are very subtle at first. Many affected bitches start by having a subtle change in their demeanor (Figure 12.5). This usually manifests as lifting a lip or growling at her puppies. This quickly progresses to facial itching or rubbing. The next stage can involve generalized muscle tremors and may progress to seizures. Before attempting treatment, bitches with any of these signs should be presented for veterinary examination or at least a call made for advice.

Blood calcium needs to be boosted quickly when hypocalcemia occurs, but this comes with other potentially severe side effects including potentially lethal cardiac arrhythmias. It therefore should always be done very carefully. Veterinarians can calibrate treatment by measuring the ionized calcium level in a blood sample. This reveals the circulating level of available calcium in the blood. Correction of a low calcium level can be accomplished in the immediate crisis by injectable or oral products. The choice between these depends on the specific situation and the degree of hypocalcemia. Any treatment should only be implemented if there is confirmation of low calcium levels and should only be done under the direction of a veterinarian. Feeding adequate stage-specific diets, as well as quickly responding to a decrease in feed intake are practices that avoid hypocalcemia, and effectively eliminate the need for treatment.

12.2.4 Metritis

Metritis is an infection of the uterus and usually occurs in the post-partum period. The usual signs are fever with a vulvar discharge that has a purulent appearance and may have a foul odor. Bitches with these signs should be examined. Metritis involves both the superficial and muscular layers of the uterus and can result in a very profound systemic infection.

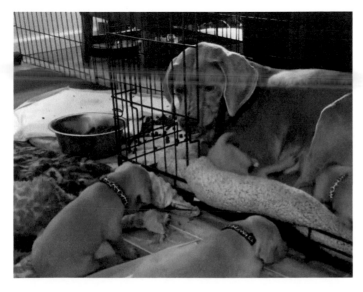

Figure 12.5 This bitch with hypocalcemia is starting to snarl at her puppies when they try to nurse. Photo by JTC.

Treatment is very similar to that for mastitis: antibiotics, anti-inflammatories, and gastro-protective agents. Noticing any changes to the lochia or to eating habits will result in quick diagnosis and effective treatment.

12.3 Care of Neonatal Puppies through Three Weeks

12.3.1 Normal Puppy Development

After puppies are born, they have many milestones they each need to reach before moving on to their new homes. Their organs and bodies still require further development and growth beyond the stage they have attained at birth. Puppies take many months or up to a few years to reach full maturity. It is essential to remember that puppies are not just miniature adult dogs because they have many metabolic differences from adult dogs that can be important factors to be considered in the management of their growth as well as in any medical interventions. Several systems within a puppy need to fully develop and then mature before that puppy reaches its full and functional maturity at adulthood. These include:

- the kidneys
- a fully competent immune system
- full ability to produce blood clotting factors
- production systems for blood cells
- the nervous system.

The differences between puppies and mature dogs means that the parameters for physical examination are different for puppies than for adults. It takes puppies several weeks to develop what would be considered normal values for an adult dog. Several basic parameters that are used to monitor health are markedly different between puppies and adults. The typical parameters are shown below.

- Body temperature range:
  - puppies 35–37°C (95–99°F)
  - adult dogs 37.5–39.2°C (99.5–102.5°F)
- Heart rate (tends to be lower in larger animals):
  - puppies: 180–200 beats per minute
  - adult dogs: 60–140 beats per minute
- Respiratory rate (depends on size, exertion, and anxiety):
  - puppies: 15–35 breaths per minute
  - adult dogs: 10–30 breaths per minute when at rest or sleeping.

Puppy brains cannot regulate body temperature until after 3 weeks of age, so environmental control of temperature is crucial during these early weeks of life. Production of any clotting factors, and therefore the ability to control any severe blood loss, is incomplete until at least 15–18 weeks of age. This is the reason behind not recommending surgery in any neonates less than 8–12 weeks of age. Careful consideration of the reason for any surgery and whether it is medically necessary should be considered carefully in all cases requiring surgical intervention.

Puppies require stimulation from the dam or a caretaker to urinate and defecate for the first couple of weeks. The dam does this by licking and nuzzling the puppy. However, severely distended bladders and colons will excrete the waste on their own, without stimulation. This spontaneous excretion is not normal and is not ideal for the puppy. Care should be taken to ensure that puppies are stimulated on a regular basis so that defecation and urination occur normally. The first feces a puppy passes are meconium, which is yellow to orange, sticky and the consistency of soft serve ice cream. After the puppy begins to process the colostrum and milk the feces become more typical in color and texture.

Puppies actively dream while sleeping. This active dream state is essential for the maturation of the nervous system and is very important for normal development. Puppies should never lie still without some form of active dreaming. Careful observation of any individual puppy that is sleeping quietly and without movement is imperative because this is an indication of a potentially severe underlying problem.

The eyes and ears of puppies open around two weeks of age, and this usually corresponds with an increase in activity level (Figure 12.6). Bedding material in the whelping box is important at this stage. It should be easily cleaned, but also needs to be of a good stable material that allows for the puppies to grip it as they enter this more active phase of development. Slippery surfaces prevent the puppies from getting on the pads of their feet. This predisposes them to "swimmers syndrome," which is a generalized flattening of the chest. Rather than being an oval from top to bottom, the chest flattens to a rectangle and compresses the internal organs. Mild cases can be treated with daily exercises, but it is best to completely avoid the situation by ensuring that the whelping box is filled with material that allows the puppies to move on their feet and not on their stomach.

The newborn puppy has an immune system that has not yet been stimulated to produce any protection against environmental organisms. At birth puppies have only a small number of antibodies (mainly in the IgG class) circulating in their bodies. Antibodies are large proteins that help to ward off infectious agents. Puppies are initially unable to produce their own antibodies.

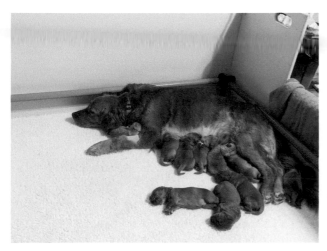

Figure 12.6 Puppies move actively and need a good floor surface to avoid leg problems. Activity levels increase dramatically in the first three weeks. Photo by Renee Machen.

They therefore depend on protection that comes from their dam (Figure 12.7). Good husbandry of the pregnant bitch usually assures a good degree of what is called "passive transfer" of immunity to the puppies. This is accomplished by the passage of antibodies through the placenta, and (at higher levels) by the first milk (colostrum) that is produced.

Vaccination of the dam ensures that these antibodies are available in adequate amounts for transfer to the puppies. If a bitch is due a booster vaccination during the pregnancy or lactation, then it is best to provide this before mating. Dams that are current on vaccination are likely to have protective levels of the antibody class IgG circulating in the blood. About 5% to 10% of these antibodies transfer through the placenta to the puppy during the last weeks of gestation.

Adequate transfer of antibodies right after birth can be accomplished in two ways:

- colostrum intake
- administration of serum from a well-vaccinated adult animal.

Antibodies from the dam's colostrum are absorbed by the gastrointestinal tract of the puppy in the first few hours of life. The puppy's gastrointestinal tract is permeable to the large IgG molecules for the first 12–15 hours of life. As much as 40% of the needed transfer occurs within the first 4 hours of life, so nursing as soon as possible is important. After 4 hours the absorption of these antibodies decreases drastically. The gastrointestinal tract is closed completely by 15 hours and can no longer serve as a portal for any antibody transfer. Normal puppies that have been born via natural delivery begin to move and search for a teat within minutes of birth. Puppies should nurse often. It is best to ensure that puppies receive adequate antibodies at birth to supplement what is available through the placenta. Colostrum, in addition to antibodies, has several other important characteristics that make it essential as a component for normal puppy development.

The antibodies that come from placental transfer or from the colostrum are the only defense the puppy possesses until its own immune system develops at around 6 to 8 weeks old.

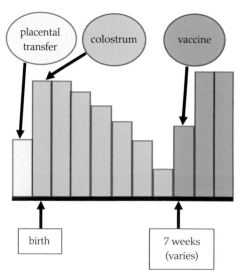

Figure 12.7 Puppies rely on immunity acquired from their dams. This is acquired across the placenta and through the ingestion of colostrum during the first few hours of life. This immunity declines to a point at which the puppy is responsive to vaccination, achieving protection with its own immune response. Figure by DPS.

At this age, the puppy can produce its own individual immune response to an infectious challenge.

Puppies that are born to dams that have no colostrum, are orphaned, or are otherwise unable to nurse effectively should be given serum from a well-vaccinated adult dog via oro-gastric intubation. Protective levels of IgG are found in neonates that receive serum orally within 4 hours of birth. It is wise to keep frozen adult serum on hand for this purpose. Alternatively, serum can be given subcutaneously (under the skin) but the levels achieved by this route are much lower than those following ingestion. The protection from subcutaneous administration is unlikely to be fully protective, even if given early in the post-partum period.

The antibodies that puppies acquire through the passive pathways of placenta and colostrum wane over time. There is a window of time between the dam's passive antibodies diminishing and the puppy's own antibodies rising during which the puppy is vulnerable to infections from which they were previously protected by their dam's contribution of antibodies. Vaccination for common diseases should begin during this time window because at that point the puppy's own immune system can mount a response and produce its own memory cells. Before this window, the dam's antibodies are in sufficient quantities to inactivate vaccines that are administered to the puppy. Waiting too long for vaccination provides a longer window of susceptibility during which puppies are vulnerable.

Unfortunately, the rate at which the maternal antibodies decline varies from puppy to puppy, but usually occurs around 7 to 8 weeks of age. This is highly variable even in individuals from a single litter. The variability in this important period is one reason that multiple vaccinations are usually recommended for puppies. Puppies with earlier decline of maternal antibodies will then be protected, even though the vaccine in their littermates with more persistent maternal antibodies will have inactivated the vaccine. Those littermates with more persistent maternal antibodies will then be stimulated and protected by the vaccinations that occur later in the series because their maternal antibodies will have then declined sufficiently for the vaccine to be effective.

Puppies that come from a dam who was not vaccinated or had an unknown background should have their first vaccination a bit earlier than the usual recommendation to provide protection in case the puppy did not get adequate antibody transfer early in life. The first vaccine is typically a combination that provides protection from canine distemper virus, adenovirus, parainfluenza and parvo virus. It is important that veterinary direction be followed to ensure that well-protected puppies are sent to their new homes.

12.3.2 Neonate Viability

Viability parameters have been established for puppies. Breeders should be aware of the parameters, their limits as to utility, and how to use these to test for any change in status of the viability of a neonate. Two methods are generally used to address viability: APGAR and reflexes. Any deficits in these two viability tests indicate a puppy that should be examined immediately.

APGAR stands for:

- appearance
- pulse

- grimace
- activity
- respiration (and neonatal reflexes).

The APGAR system for dogs has been adapted from the human scoring system that uses the same name (Table 12.1). This rating system incorporates:

- heart rate
- respiratory effort, rate, and vocalizing
- irritability reflex
- motility
- mucous membrane color.

These parameters are scored, and a total score yields an estimate of overall puppy vigor. Most normal puppies will score seven or greater. Puppies from the brachycephalic breeds tend to have relatively lower viability scores after birth, so there is an adapted scale just for those breeds. However, brachycephalic puppies tend to score just as high as other breeds if the dam is not stressed at the time of a caesarian section. Judicious use of drugs prior to delivery and care of the neonates can help to minimize any adverse effects in brachycephalic breeds.

The other system that can be used to assess viability is the evaluation of neonatal reflexes. Reflexes should be checked once daily on each puppy. These include three parameters: rooting, righting, and suckling.

Rooting is determined by making a shelf with a hand or fist just in front of the puppy's nose to evaluate whether they push up against the hand as if they were seeking a nipple. Righting consists of gently placing the puppy on its back and seeing if it will turn itself over (Figure 12.8). Suckling is evaluated by placing a finger in the mouth of a puppy to assure that it will attempt to nurse. Puppies with delayed or non-existent reflexes warrant examination.

Table 12.1 The APGAR system for neonatal puppies has been adapted from the one used for human neonates.

Canine APGAR Scoring System			
Parameter	Score		
	0	1	2
heart rate in beats per minute	less than 180	180–220	greater than 220
respiratory effort and respiratory rate per minute	no crying	mild crying	active crying
	less than 6 per min.	6–15 per min.	over 15 per min.
irritability reflex	absent	grimace	vigorous
motility	flaccid	some flexion	active motion
mucous membrane color	cyanotic (blue)	pale (white)	pink

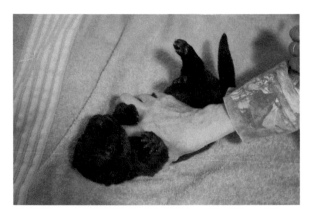

Figure 12.8 Righting reflexes can be checked by gently placing a puppy on its back. Photo by Jill Keaton.

12.3.3 Neonate Mortality

Even with the best management, not all puppies survive. Rates of neonatal mortality range from 2% to 30%. Around 50% of neonatal deaths occur within the first 3 to 5 days after birth.

Neonatal puppies can die from several infectious diseases and from traumatic injuries. In addition to these two general sources of loss are three other threats that are inherently limited to the neonatal period (Figure 12.9). These three can each quickly compromise a neonate severely enough that it can die if no treatment is offered:

- hypothermia (low body temperature)
- hypovolemia (low blood volume)
- hypoglycemia (low blood sugar).

These are known as the three "Hs" and all management should be directed at avoiding these conditions so that they do not need to be corrected by interventions. All breeders and veterinarians need to address each of these when confronted with a neonate that is failing to thrive.

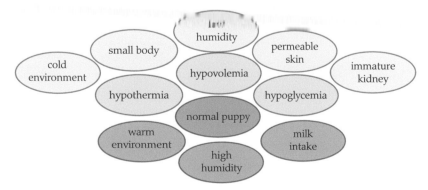

Figure 12.9 Normal puppies depend on a good and supportive environment. Increasing the level of any of several threats can make them susceptible to the three Hs. Figure by DPS.

Each of the three Hs occurs because of several interacting factors that are unique to this early period of life. Several details of puppy anatomy and physiology combine to make temperature and fluid balance difficult. Puppies are small and have a high skin surface area to body volume ratio that facilitates fluid loss. Puppy skin is highly permeable, facilitating the loss of water through evaporation into the environment. In addition, puppy kidneys are immature and are inefficient at regulating internal hydration. Environmental control of heat and humidity in the whelping area can greatly help to offset these challenges. Keeping the room warm, at temperatures of least 24°C (75°F), as well as providing a humidity around 50% should assist in preventing environmental dehydration in the first few weeks. Compromised neonates or those that are not doing as well as their littermates may need special accommodations with increased warmth and humidity.

Hypothermia is the first "H." At birth all puppies are thrust from the very humid and warm environment in the uterus into an oxygen-deprived, cold, and dehydrating environment. This is a detriment to the puppies right from the very start because puppies are made up of 80% water. Their small body size is associated with a relatively large surface area, and loss of heat into a cold environment can be rapid and irreversible. Cold puppies need to be warmed quickly enough to stabilize them but slowly enough to avoid overheating them.

Hypovolemia can be a consequence of the neonate's inability to concentrate fluids due to incomplete function of their still-developing kidneys. A puppy's body rapidly metabolizes any fluid and nutrients that are ingested. The high water content of puppies couples with their high metabolic rate to equate to a need for them to be fed frequently. All neonates should be eating at least every hour to two hours. The best indicator of hydration status is weight. All puppies should be weighed at birth, prior to their first nursing session. This birth weight is important in determining daily weight gain as well as helping to identify any puppies that are falling behind and need supplementation.

Some litters will have a loss in weight within the first day. This is considered normal by some experts, but the best evidence shows that normal puppies maintain or gain weight within the first 24 hours. All puppies should gain a target of 5–10% of their birth weight daily. Daily gains in bodyweight in the range of 5–12% are considered normal. Inadequate weight gain is true of any puppy with a plateau in weight for 24 hours or a loss of more than 4–10% of weight from one day to the next. Puppies losing weight are at risk for several health complications and possible death. Puppies that are 25% lighter than their littermates are deemed "high risk" and should be watched very carefully (Figure 12.10).

Hypoglycemia is a low blood sugar level. Blood sugar (glucose) is essential for puppies to maintain normal organ metabolism. As puppies have a rapid metabolism, hypoglycemia in puppies is acutely life-threatening. Normal puppies nurse, fall off the teat and actively sleep, then wake up and nurse again. They do this frequently throughout both day and night. All puppies should have the opportunity to free nurse. If hand reared, they should be fed every 1 to 2 hours for the first two weeks of life. Weak or inactive puppies should be noted and examined by a veterinarian.

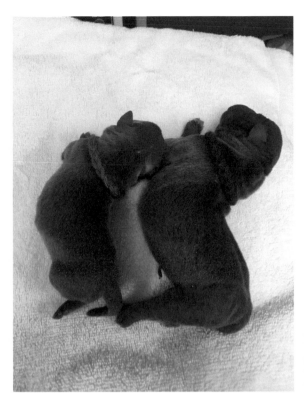

Figure 12.10 The smaller of these two puppies is a "high risk" individual and should be watched carefully to assure that it is gaining weight. Photo by JTC.

12.4 Supplemental Nutritional Support

Puppies that are not gaining weight appropriately, or those that have an identified problem, may benefit from supplemental feeding (Figure 12.11). This can be accomplished in three ways:

- graft the puppy on to another dam
- have the puppy nurse without competition
- supplement with artificial milk replacer.

Grafting is placing the puppy with a lactating bitch that has puppies of a similar size, but that has only a few puppies of her own so has the capacity for sufficient milk production to support the additional puppy. Grafting should be approached with caution as not all bitches will accept a puppy from another litter. Rejection may occur suddenly and violently. Despite this potential detraction, grafting is advantageous because it provides a natural source of milk, as well as allowing a natural interval for nursing. It also allows for normal socialization. It is more convenient than other approaches because once the initial grafting is accomplished no intervention is required on the part of the breeder.

Removing competition from a small puppy involves allowing it to nurse on its dam alone without having to compete for a nipple with its stronger littermates. This can be a simple way to supplement but should only be used for puppies that have an intact, strong

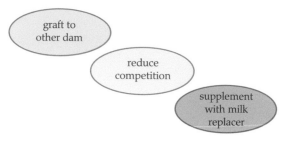

Figure 12.11 The different methods of supplementing a puppy have very different requirements for action on the part of caretakers. This can influence the practicality of which method to choose. Figure by DPS.

suckle reflex and that are well enough to nurse on their own. This must be done multiple times a day, although it is usually true that the puppy is getting at least some opportunity for nursing in between the sessions when competition has been removed.

Nutrition can also be provided by supplementation with artificial milk replacer and through artificial feeding. Milk replacer for puppies varies as widely as the diets available to feed adults. All breeders need to consider if supplementation is necessary and the risks that supplementation may carry for the individual puppy. Two main concerns are the nutritional content of the replacer, and the possibility of aspiration of milk replacer into the puppy's lungs. There are no products currently available that are canine in origin, so breeders need to find what is commercially available to them and then decide what is the best choice for their specific situation. Cow and goat milk are not similar in composition to canine milk but can be sufficient when needed. Despite the variability of commercial products, these are still greatly superior to homemade products. Homemade formulas are difficult to mix appropriately, may not be balanced, and are difficult to adjust for water content.

The actual feeding of milk replacer can be achieved in many different ways. The two most commonly used methods are orogastric tube feeding and bottle feeding. The safest method to use to provide supplement is via orogastric intubation (Figure 12.12). This is the preferred method for all severely compromised neonates that have a weak suckle reflex. A tube is placed in the mouth and directed down the esophagus into the stomach. This procedure actually carries the least risk of complications because there are fail-safe ways by which to ensure that the tube is in the stomach and not in the lungs. A veterinarian or veterinary technician can easily teach a breeder how to safely perform this method. After learning the technique, a person should be able to feed a whole litter of 8 to 12 puppies

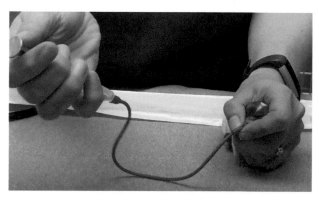

Figure 12.12 The skill of tube-feeding puppies is rapidly mastered and provides a quick and safe way to assure that puppies are getting the nutrition they need for a good start. Photo by JTC.

via orogastric tube in less than 15 to 20 minutes. This method is much preferred due to the minimal risk of aspiration of milk into the lungs.

The other method that can be used to artificially supplement is bottle feeding. This carries a greater risk of aspiration because the puppies are suckling from nipples that were designed for another species, so the size and shape are wrong. The nipples on bottles also have a higher flow than is true of the flow from the dam and can outpace a neonate's ability to swallow. Bottle feeding should only be done when the neonate has a strong suckle reflex. The best nipple to use is one designed for premature human babies and that is rated as having the slowest flow rate. This type of nipple provides the slowest flow of milk, while still allowing for natural nursing behaviour. Even with this sort of nipple there is still a higher risk of aspiration than occurs with tube feeding. Any other types of supplemental feeding should be avoided.

All supplementations should be done under the direction of a veterinarian and should be accompanied by daily weight checks. Supplementation may lead to rapid weight gain. This can predispose the puppies to obesity. Caution must be used to ensure the puppies are not gaining more than 10–15% of their body weight daily. Once the puppies are three weeks old a gruel can be introduced as they transition from milk to dog food (Figure 12.13). This can be done with their intended puppy food, soaked to a watery consistency and offered several times a day. As the puppies mature and learn to use their mouths to prehend the food the water content can be gradually lowered.

12.5 Neonate Neurologic Stimulation

Breeders can help to stimulate neurologic growth in puppies during the first 3 weeks of life. This can be accomplished with a few exercises and experiences that can start as early as day 3 after birth. The "Bio Sensor" or "Super Dog" program was developed by the US military as an attempt to improve the performance of their military working dogs. They found that dogs benefitted by implementing five different exercises once daily from days 3 to 16. These simple exercises should not be used in place of normal socialization that a breeder performs during the early stages of life but should instead be used as a supplement to the

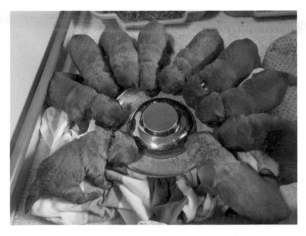

Figure 12.13 Puppies can be introduced to gruel as they gain mobility and activity. Photo by Renee Machen.

normal daily routine. Observations over six months revealed that puppies not receiving this stimulation performed equally well as those that have been stimulated with a targeted program. The program therefore provides a somewhat temporary advantage, which indicates that general normal socialization is just as important as targeted stimulation.

New scents can be introduced to puppies intended for scent work. Exposure to new scents can be started when puppies are 3 to 5 days old. They can be exposed once daily, and only for a few seconds. The scents can be changed every few days. Essential oils and other non-toxic substances are preferred as the sources of the scents. These exercises stimulate the developing neurologic system and support growth and maturation of the puppies.

12.6 Key Points

- Uterine involution is a process that takes several weeks.
- Lochial discharge is normal during uterine involution.
- Lactation is metabolically demanding, and the dam's nutritional needs must be met.
- Colostrum is the "first milk" and is rich in antibodies that protect the neonate.
- Mastitis can be managed best following early detection.
- Hypocalcemia is most common in heavy lactation and can be avoided by careful and wise management of calcium nutrition.
- Metritis is inflammation of the uterus and is managed by antibiotics.
- Puppies are prone to hypothermia, hypovolemia, and hypoglycemia, and these can be managed by diligent feeding management.
- Puppies are born without immunity and gain their first immunity through the placenta and colostrum.
- Immunity from the dam wanes over time, and at that point puppies need vaccinations.
- Puppies can be deliberately stimulated to enhance their development.

Index